The Physiotherapist's Pocket Book

To Jack

For Churchill Livingstone:

Senior commissioning editor: Heidi Allen
Project development manager: Dinah Thom
Project manager: Joannah Duncan
Designer: Judith Wright
Illustration manager: Bruce Hogarth

The Physiotherapist's Pocket Book

ESSENTIAL FACTS AT YOUR FINGERTIPS

Jonathan Kenyon BSc MCSP

Senior Physiotherapist, Guy's and St Thomas's Hospital NHS Trust, London, UK

Karen Kenyon BSc BA MCSP

Senior Physiotherapist, St George's Hospital Healthcare NHS Trust, London, UK

CHURCHILL LIVINGSTONE

EDINBURGH LONDON NEW YORK OXFORD PHILADELPHIA ST LOUIS SYDNEY TORONTO 2004

CHURCHILL LIVINGSTONE
An imprint of Elsevier Limited

First published 2004
Reprinted 2004, 2005

ISBN 0 443 07318 X

British Library Cataloguing in Publication Data
A catalogue record for this book is available from the British Library

Library of Congress Cataloguing in Publication Data
A catalogue record for this book is available from the Library of Congress

Note
Medical knowledge is constantly changing. As new information becomes available, changes in treatment, procedures, equipment and the use of drugs become necessary. The author, contributor and the publishers have, as far as it is possible, taken care to ensure that the information given in this text is accurate and up to date. However, readers are strongly advised to confirm that the information, especially with regard to drug usage, complies with the latest legislation and standards of practice.

Neither the publishers nor the author will be liable for any loss or damage of any nature occasioned to or suffered by any person acting or refraining from acting as a result of reliance on the material contained in this publication.

The Publisher

Printed in China
C/03

Contents

Section 2 Neurology 117

Section 3 Respiratory 159

Section 4 Pharmacology 209

Section 5 Appendices 233

Inside back cover

Preface

The idea for this book developed while we were students. As much as we would try to remember all the tests, normal values, pathologies, contraindications, anatomy, etc., there were times while on clinical placements when we needed to check something but did not have textbooks to hand. The solution was simple. Before going on placement we'd prepare pocket-sized reference notes that we could carry around and access quickly. Over a period of time, we found we had developed a compendium of useful information covering all the core areas of physiotherapy. This remained useful when we were newly qualified and rotating from one specialization to another every few months. Our intention in producing this book has been to provide all this information in one handy reference that can be used during clinical practice.

The sections within this book cover the core areas of physiotherapy – musculoskeletal, neurology and respiratory. There is also a section on pharmacology and eight appendices. It is beyond the scope and size of the book to cover all the specialist areas, but we hope that the chapters are broad enough to be useful to everyone. We have tried to include as much information as possible by using illustrations, charts, tables and lists wherever practicable. This book does not take the place of a textbook but is a handy, pocket-sized collection of essential facts and figures that you can carry with you anywhere.

Jonathan and Karen Kenyon
London, 2004

Acknowledgements

Taking on a project like this would be impossible without the input from a large number of people. Some gave us the confidence to get started, while others provided guidance. Some checked what we had compiled and others were always there when the long evenings and weekends took their toll. To all of those people, we would like to extend our heartfelt thanks.

In particular we would like to thank our colleagues at Guy's and St Thomas's and St George's Hospitals for their continued support and encouragement throughout this project. Special thanks go to John Hammond, Sally Paterson, Sandy Chambers, Gareth Jones, Joanna McIlmurray, Bruce Paton, Tanya Usher and Ruth McGuinness who so generously gave up their time to read and comment on the various sections of this book.

We would also like to offer our sincere appreciation to Professor John Trounce for reviewing the pharmacology section, Sheila Kitchen for her kind advice and encouragement, Nicola Petty for her feedback and late night e-mails, and Christine Bithell for seeing the value in our idea and steering us towards a publisher.

Finally we would like to thank our friends ... for being just that. And our families, for believing in us from the start.

SECTION 1

Musculoskeletal

SECTION 1

Musculoskeletal anatomy illustrations

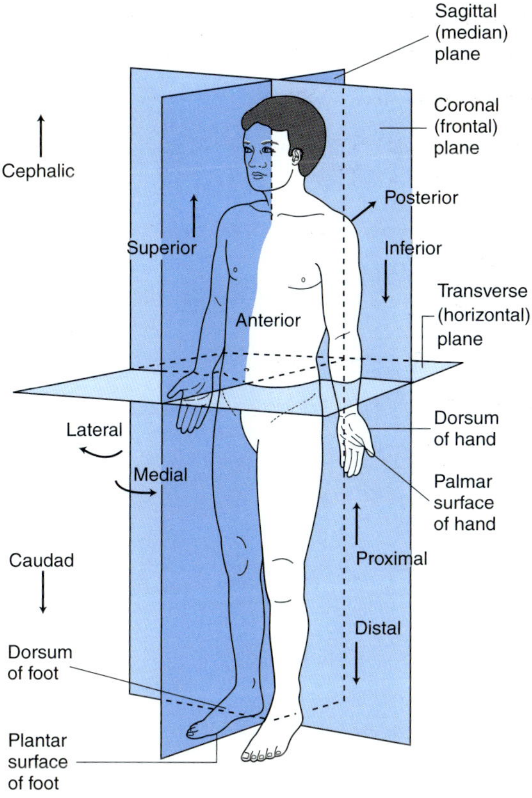

Figure 1.1 Anatomical position showing cardinal planes and directional terminology.

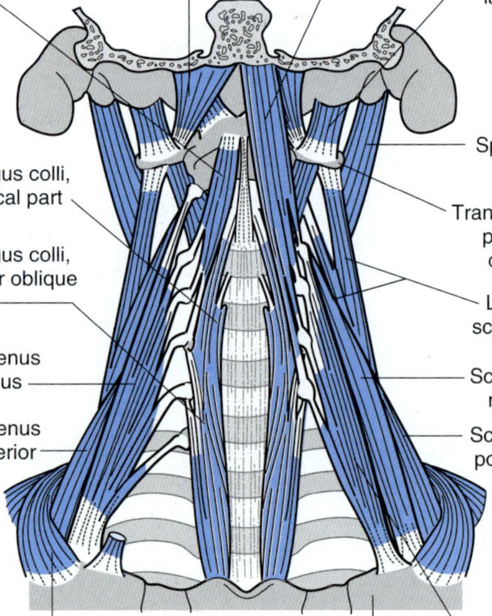

Figure 1.2 Anterior and lateral muscles of the neck.

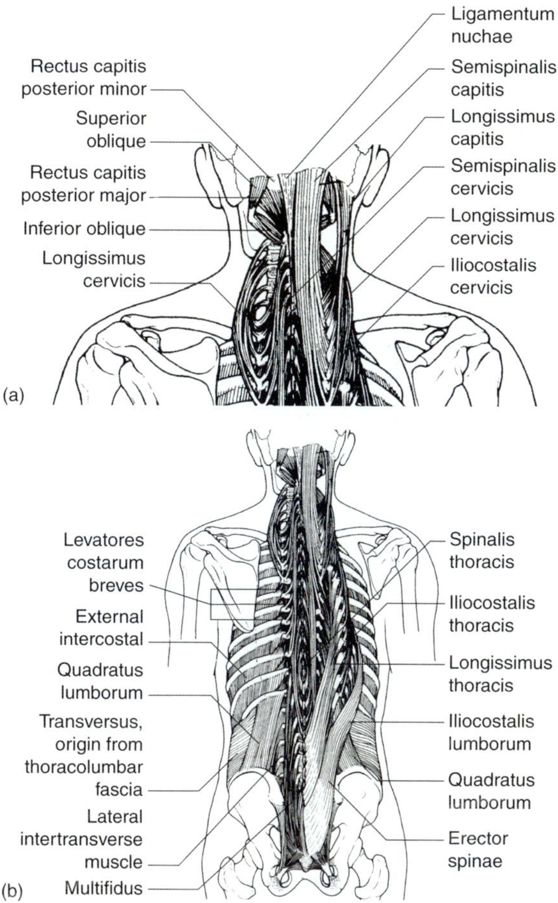

Figure 1.3 Deep muscles of the back.

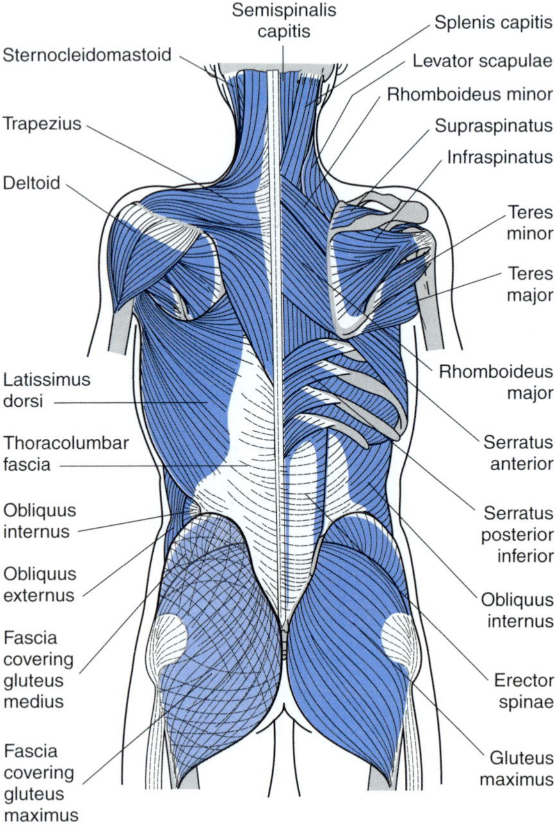

Figure 1.4 Superficial muscles of the back, neck and trunk.

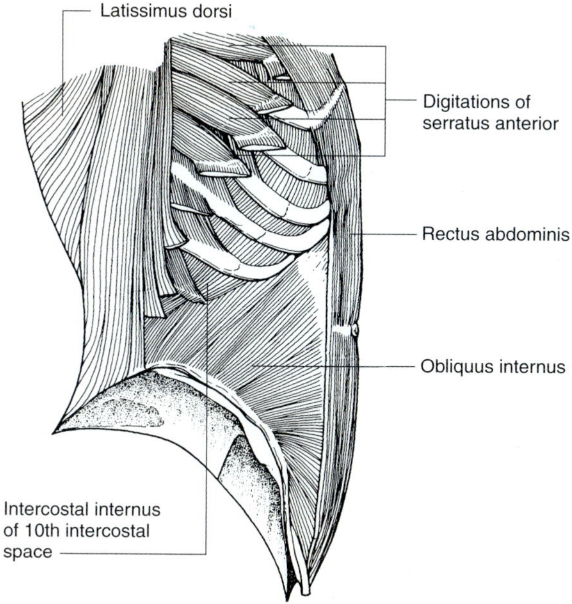

Figure 1.5 Muscles of the right side of the trunk.

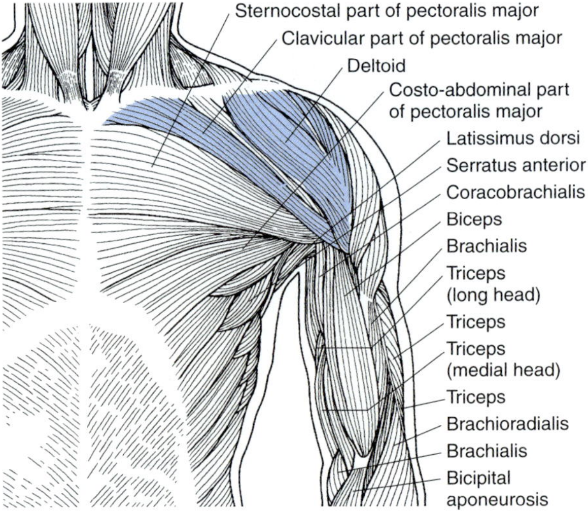

Figure 1.6 Superficial muscles of the anterior chest and arm. Left side.

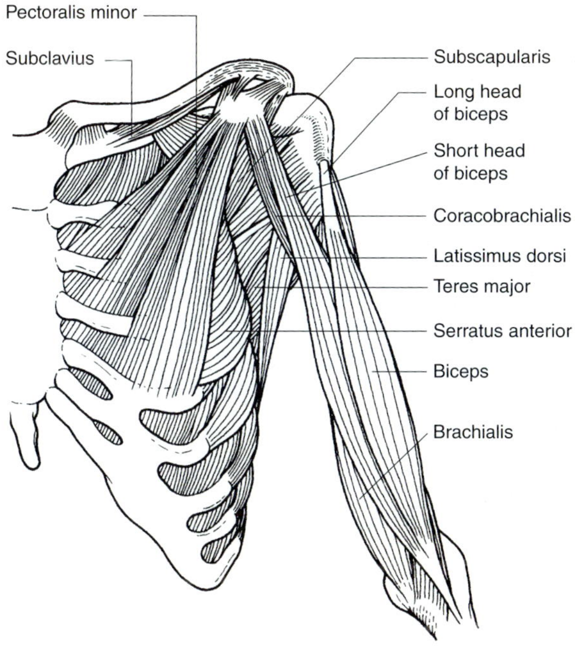

Figure 1.7 Deep muscles of the anterior chest and upper arm. Left side.

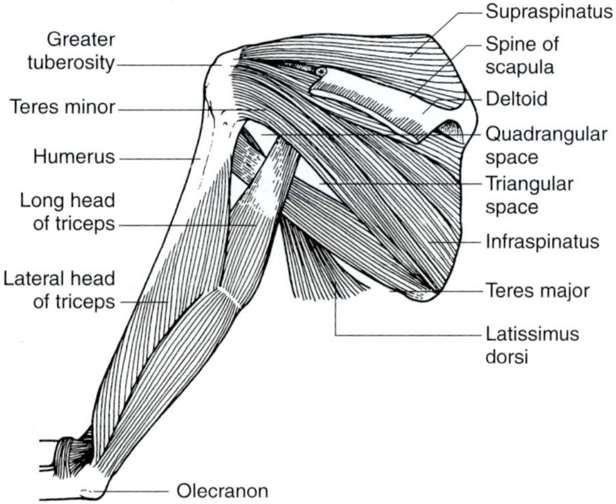

Figure 1.8 Muscles of the posterior scapula and upper arm. Left side.

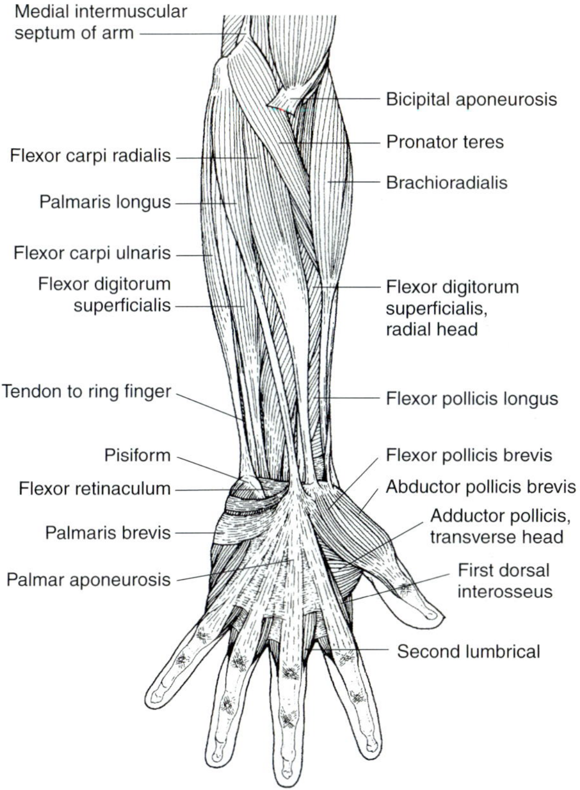

Figure 1.9 Superficial flexors of the left forearm.

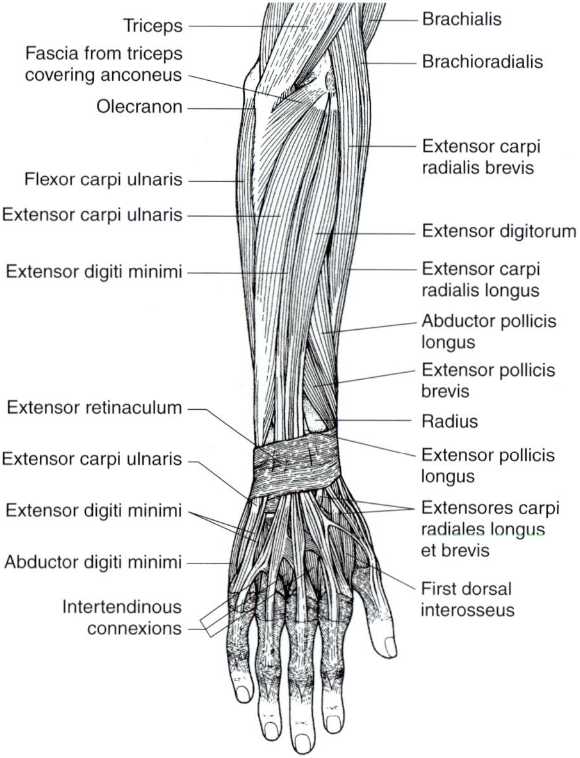

Figure 1.10 Superficial extensors of the right forearm.

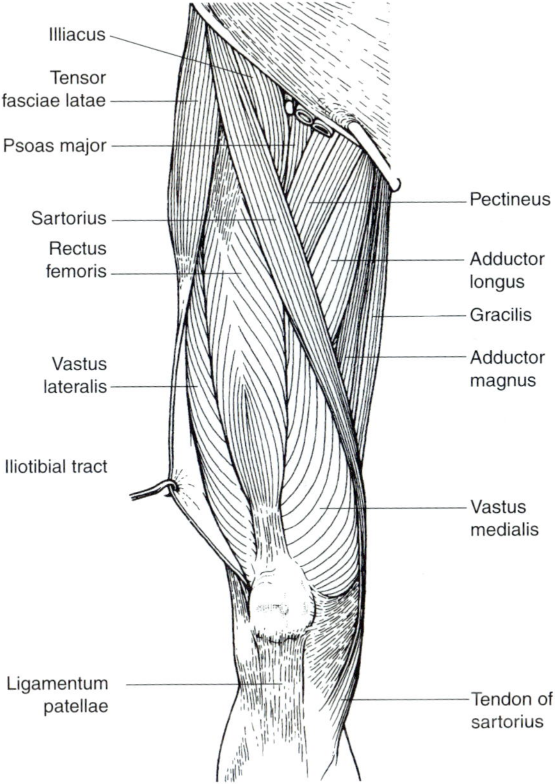

Figure 1.11 Superficial muscles of the anterior right thigh.

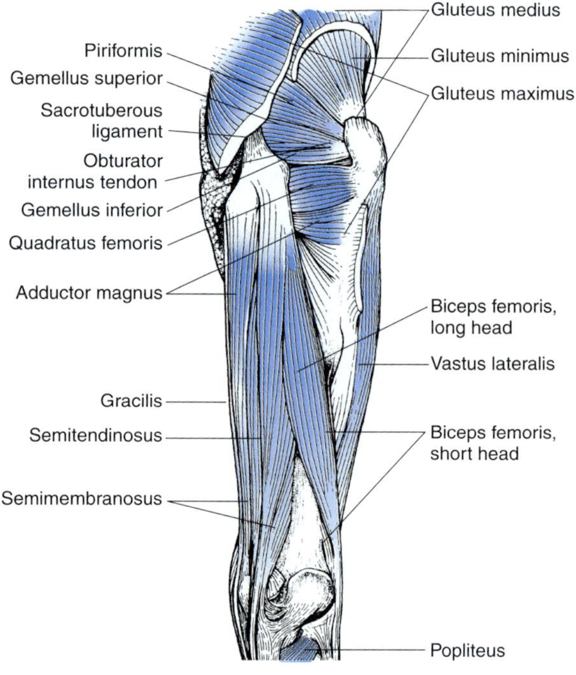

Figure 1.12 Muscles of the posterior right thigh.

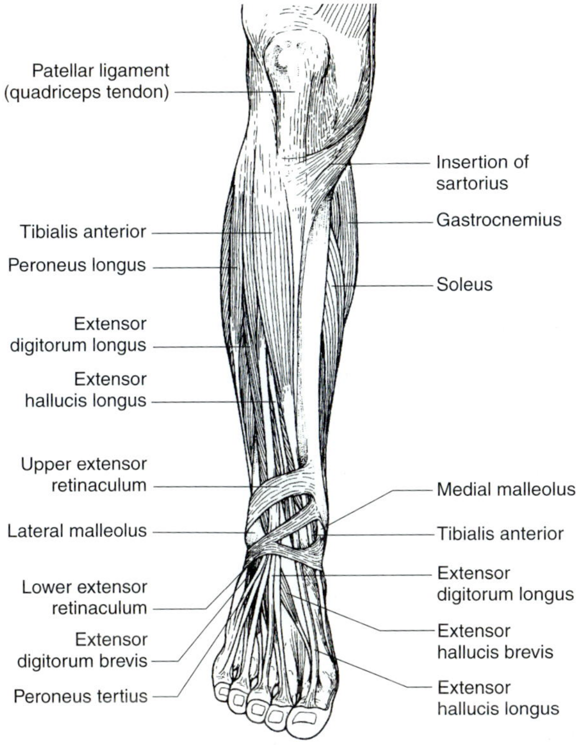

Figure 1.13 Muscles of the anterior right leg.

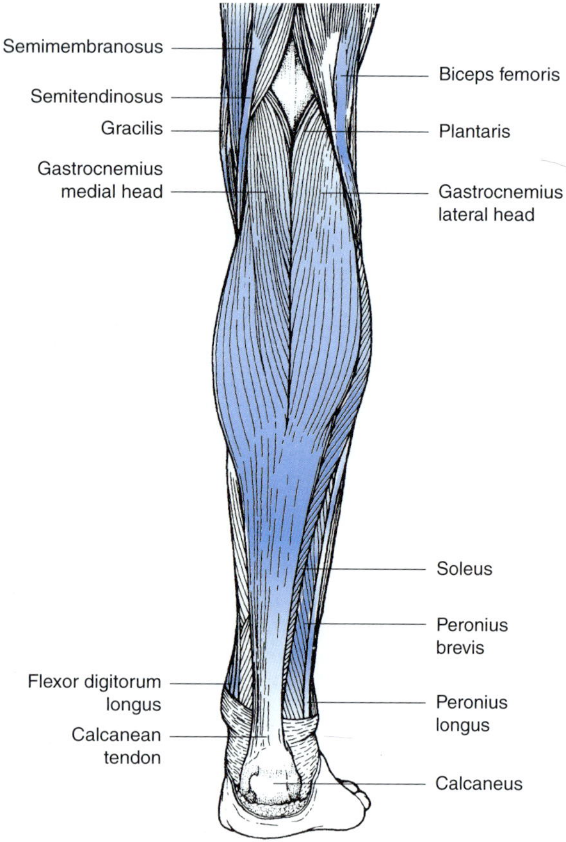

Figure 1.14 Superficial muscles of the posterior right calf.

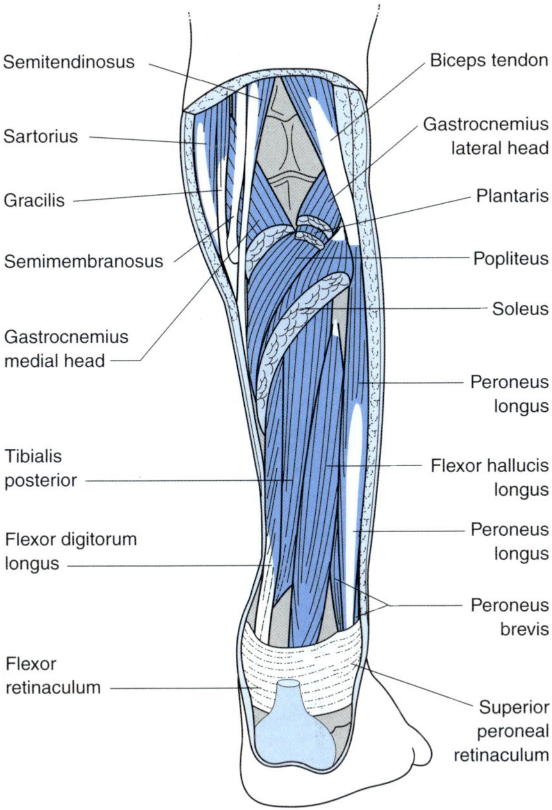

Figure 1.15 Deep muscles of the posterior right calf.

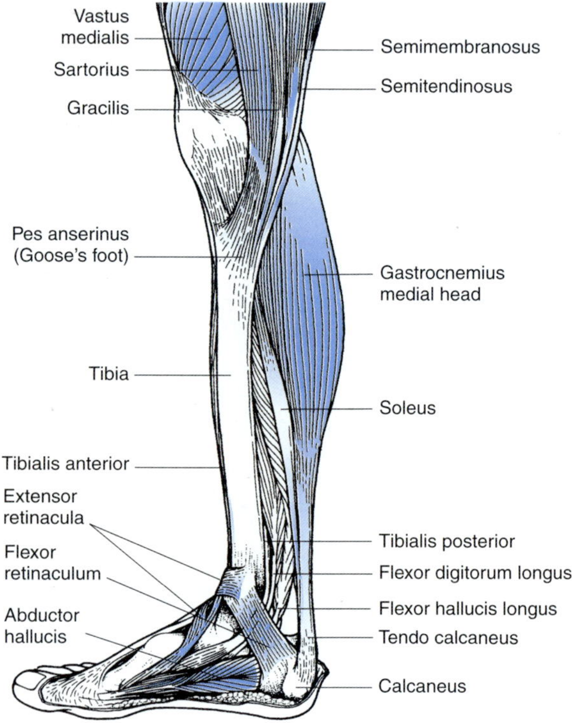

Figure 1.16 Muscles of the medial right leg.

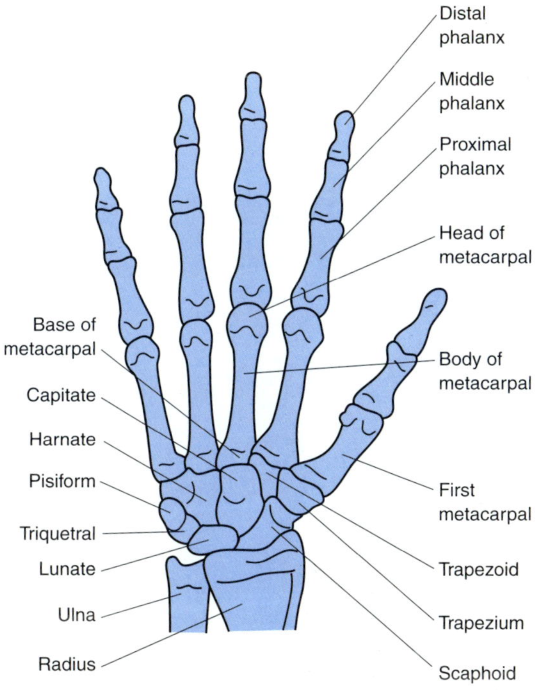

Figure 1.17 Bones of the right hand.

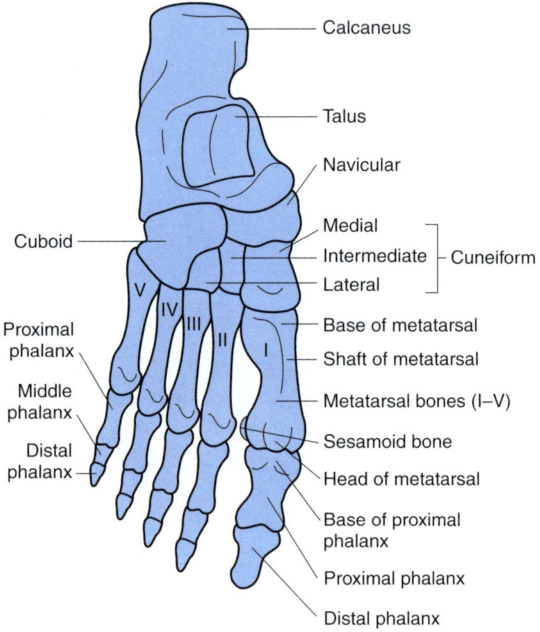

Figure 1.18 Bones of the right foot.

Muscles listed by function

Head and neck

Flexors: longus colli, longus capitis, rectus capitis anterior, sternocleidomastoid, scalenus anterior

Lateral flexors: erector spinae, rectus capitis lateralis, scalenes (anterior, medius and posterior), splenius cervicis, splenius capitis, trapezius, levator scapulae, sternocleidomastoid

Extensors: levator scapulae, splenius cervicis, trapezius, splenius capitis, semispinalis, superior oblique, sternocleidomastoid, erector spinae, rectus capitis posterior major, rectus capitis posterior minor

Rotators: semispinalis, multifidus, scalenus anterior, splenius cervicis, sternocleidomastoid, splenius capitis, rectus capitis posterior major, inferior oblique

Trunk

Flexors: rectus abdominis, external oblique, internal oblique, psoas minor, psoas major, iliacus

Rotators: multifidus, rotatores, semispinalis, internal oblique, external oblique

Lateral flexors: quadratus lumborum, intertransversarii, external oblique, internal oblique, erector spinae, multifidus

Extensors: quadratus lumborum, multifidus, semispinalis, erector spinae, interspinales, rotatores

Scapula

Retractors: rhomboid minor, rhomboid major, trapezius, levator scapulae

Protractors: serratus anterior, pectoralis minor

Elevators: trapezius, levator scapulae

Depressors: trapezius

Lateral rotators: trapezius, serratus anterior

Medial rotators: rhomboid major, rhomboid minor, pectoralis minor, levator scapulae

Shoulder

Flexors: pectoralis major, deltoid (anterior fibres), biceps brachii (long head), coracobrachialis

Extensors: latissimus dorsi, teres major, pectoralis major, deltoid (posterior fibres), triceps (long head)

Abductors: supraspinatus, deltoid (middle fibres)

Adductors: coracobrachialis, pectoralis major, latissimus dorsi, teres major
Medial rotators: subscapularis, teres major, latissimus dorsi, pectoralis major, deltoid (anterior fibres)
Lateral rotators: teres minor, infraspinatus, deltoid (posterior fibres)

Elbow

Flexors: biceps brachii, brachialis, brachioradialis, pronator teres
Extensors: triceps brachii, anconeus
Pronators: pronator teres, pronator quadratus
Supinators: supinator, biceps brachii

Wrist

Flexors: flexor carpi ulnaris, flexor carpi radialis, palmaris longus, flexor digitorum superficialis, flexor digitorum profundus, flexor pollicis longus
Extensors: extensor carpi radialis longus, extensor carpi radialis brevis, extensor carpi ulnaris, extensor digitorum, extensor indicis, extensor digiti minimi, extensor pollicis longus, extensor pollicis brevis
Ulnar deviation: flexor carpi ulnaris, extensor carpi ulnaris
Radial deviation: flexor carpi radialis, extensor carpi radialis longus, extensor carpi radialis brevis, abductor pollicis longus, extensor pollicis longus, extensor pollicis brevis

Fingers

Flexors: flexor digitorum superficialis, flexor digitorum profundus, lumbricals, flexor digiti minimi brevis
Extensors: extensor digitorum, extensor digiti minimi, extensor indicis, interossei, lumbricals
Abductors: dorsal interossei, abductor digiti minimi, opponens digiti minimi
Adductors: palmar interossei

Thumb

Flexors: flexor pollicis longus, flexor pollicis brevis
Extensors: extensor pollicis longus, extensor pollicis brevis, abductor pollicis longus
Abductors: abductor pollicis longus, abductor pollicis brevis
Adductors: adductor pollicis
Opposition: opponens pollicis

Hip

Flexors: psoas major, iliacus, rectus femoris, sartorius, pectineus
Extensors: gluteus maximus, semitendinosus, semimembranosus, biceps femoris
Abductors: gluteus maximus, gluteus medius, gluteus minimus, tensor fascia lata, sartorius, piriformis
Adductors: adductor magnus, adductor longus, adductor brevis, gracilis, pectineus
Medial rotators: gluteus medius, gluteus minimus, tensor fascia lata
Lateral rotators: gluteus maximus, piriformis, obturator internus, gemellus superior, gemellus inferior, quadratus femoris, obturator externus, sartorius

Knee

Flexors: semitendinosus, semimembranosus, biceps femoris, gastrocnemius, gracilis, sartorius, plantaris, popliteus
Extensors: rectus femoris, vastus lateralis, vastus intermedius, vastus medialis, tensor fascia lata
Tibial lateral rotators: biceps femoris
Tibial medial rotators: semitendinosus, semimembranosus, gracilis, sartorius, popliteus

Ankle

Plantarflexors: gastrocnemius, soleus, plantaris, peroneus longus, tibialis posterior, flexor digitorum longus, flexor hallucis longus, peroneus brevis

Dorsiflexors: tibialis anterior, extensor digitorum longus, extensor hallucis longus, peroneus tertius
Invertors: tibialis anterior, tibialis posterior
Evertors: peroneus longus, peroneus tertius, peroneus brevis

Toes

Flexors: flexor digitorum longus, flexor digitorum accessorius, flexor digitorum brevis, flexor hallucis longus, flexor hallucis brevis, flexor digiti minimi brevis, interossei, lumbricals, abductor hallucis
Extensors: extensor hallucis longus, extensor digitorum longus, extensor digitorum brevis, lumbricals, interossei
Abductors: abductor hallucis, abductor digiti minimi, dorsal interossei
Adductors: adductor hallucis, plantar interossei

Alphabetical listing of muscles

Abductor digiti minimi (foot)

Action: abducts fifth toe
Origin: calcaneal tuberosity, plantar aponeurosis, intermuscular septum
Insertion: lateral side of base of proximal phalanx of fifth toe
Nerve: lateral plantar nerve (S1–S3)

Abductor digiti minimi (hand)

Action: abducts little finger
Origin: pisiform, tendon of flexor carpi ulnaris, pisohamate ligament
Insertion: ulnar side of base of proximal phalanx of little finger
Nerve: ulnar nerve (C8, T1)

Abductor hallucis

Action: abducts and flexes great toe
Origin: flexor retinaculum, calcaneal tuberosity, plantar aponeurosis, intermuscular septum
Insertion: medial side of base of proximal phalanx of great toe
Nerve: medial plantar nerve (S1, S2)

Abductor pollicis brevis

Action: abducts thumb
Origin: flexor retinaculum, tubercles of scaphoid and trapezium, tendon of abductor pollicis longus
Insertion: radial side of base of proximal phalanx of thumb
Nerve: median nerve (C8, T1)

Abductor pollicis longus

Action: abducts and extends thumb, abducts wrist
Origin: upper part of posterior surface of ulna, middle third of posterior surface of radius, interosseous membrane
Insertion: radial side of first metacarpal base, trapezium
Nerve: posterior interosseous nerve (C7, C8)

Adductor brevis

Action: adducts hip
Origin: external aspect of body and inferior ramus of pubis
Insertion: upper half of linea aspera
Nerve: obturator nerve (L2, L3)

Adductor hallucis

Action: adducts great toe
Origin: oblique head – bases of second to fourth metatarsal, sheath of peroneus longus tendon; transverse head – plantar metatarsophalangeal ligaments of lateral three toes
Insertion: lateral side of base of proximal phalanx of great toe
Nerve: lateral plantar nerve (S2, S3)

Adductor longus

Action: adducts thigh
Origin: front of pubis
Insertion: middle third of linea aspera
Nerve: anterior division of obturator nerve (L2–L4)

Adductor magnus

Action: adducts thigh
Origin: inferior ramus of pubis, conjoined ischial ramus, inferolateral aspect of ischial tuberosity
Insertion: linea aspera, proximal part of medial supracondylar line
Nerve: obturator nerve and tibial division of sciatic nerve (L2–L4)

Adductor pollicis

Action: adducts thumb
Origin: oblique head – palmar ligaments of carpus, flexor carpi radialis tendon, base of second to fourth metacarpals, capitate; transverse head – palmar surface of third metacarpal
Insertion: base of proximal phalanx of thumb
Nerve: ulnar nerve (C8, T1)

Anconeus

Action: extends elbow
Origin: posterior surface of lateral epicondyle of humerus
Insertion: lateral surface of olecranon, upper quarter of posterior surface of ulna
Nerve: radial nerve (C6–C8)

Biceps brachii

Action: flexes shoulder and elbow, supinates forearm
Origin: long head – supraglenoid tubercle of scapula and glenoid labrum; short head – apex of coracoid process
Insertion: posterior part of radial tuberosity, bicipital aponeurosis into deep fascia over common flexor origin
Nerve: musculocutaneous nerve (C5, C6)

Biceps femoris

Action: flexes knee and extends hip, laterally rotates tibia on femur
Origin: long head – ischial tuberosity, sacrotuberous ligament; short head – lower half of lateral lip of linea aspera, lateral supracondylar line of femur, lateral intermuscular septum
Insertion: head of fibula, lateral tibial condyle
Nerve: sciatic nerve (L5–S2). Long head – tibial division; short head – common peroneal division

Brachialis

Action: flexes elbow
Origin: lower half of anterior surface of humerus, intermuscular septum
Insertion: coronoid process and tuberosity of ulna
Nerve: musculocutaneous nerve (C5, C6), radial nerve (C7)

Brachioradialis

Action: flexes elbow
Origin: upper two-thirds of lateral supracondylar ridge of humerus, lateral intermuscular septum
Insertion: lateral side of radius above styloid process
Nerve: radial nerve (C5, C6)

Coracobrachialis

Action: adducts shoulder and acts as weak flexor
Origin: apex of coracoid process
Insertion: midway along medial border of humerus
Nerve: musculocutaneous nerve (C5–C7)

Deltoid

Action: anterior fibres – flex and medially rotate shoulder; middle fibres – abduct shoulder; posterior fibres – extend and laterally rotate shoulder

Origin: anterior fibres – anterior border of lateral third of clavicle; middle fibres – lateral margin of acromion process; posterior fibres – lower edge of crest of spine of scapula
Insertion: deltoid tuberosity of humerus
Nerve: axillary nerve (C5, C6)

Diaphragm

Action: draws central tendon inferiorly. Changes volume and pressure of thoracic and abdominal cavities
Origin: posterior surface of xiphoid process, lower six costal cartilages and adjoining ribs on each side, medial and lateral arcuate ligaments, anterolateral aspect of bodies of lumbar vertebrae
Insertion: central tendon
Nerve: phrenic nerves (C3–5)

Dorsal interossei (foot)

Action: abducts toes, flexes metatarsophalangeal joints
Origin: proximal half of sides of adjacent metatarsals
Insertion: bases of proximal phalanges and dorsal digital expansion (first attaches medially to second toe; second, third and fourth attach laterally to second, third and fourth toes respectively)
Nerve: lateral plantar nerve (S2, S3)

Dorsal interossei (hand)

Action: abducts index, middle and ring fingers, flexes metacarpophalangeal joints and extends interphalangeal joints
Origin: adjacent sides of two metacarpal bones (four bipennate muscles)
Insertion: bases of proximal phalanges and dorsal digital expansions (first attaches laterally to index finger; second and third attach to both sides of middle finger; fourth attaches medially to ring finger)
Nerve: ulnar nerve (C8, T1)

Erector spinae

See iliocostalis, longissimus and spinalis

Extensor carpi radialis brevis

Action: extends and abducts wrist
Origin: lateral epicondyle via common extensor tendon
Insertion: posterior surface of base of third metacarpal
Nerve: posterior interosseous branch of radial nerve (C7, C8)

Extensor carpi radialis longus

Action: extends and abducts wrist
Origin: lower third of lateral supracondylar ridge of humerus, intermuscular septa
Insertion: posterior surface of base of second metacarpal
Nerve: radial nerve (C6, C7)

Extensor carpi ulnaris

Action: extends and adducts wrist
Origin: lateral epicondyle via common extensor tendon
Insertion: medial side of fifth metacarpal base
Nerve: posterior interosseous nerve (C7, C8)

Extensor digiti minimi

Action: extends fifth digit and wrist
Origin: lateral epicondyle via common extensor tendon, intermuscular septa
Insertion: dorsal digital expansion of fifth digit
Nerve: posterior interosseous nerve (C7, C8)

Extensor digitorum

Action: extends fingers and wrist
Origin: lateral epicondyle via common extensor tendon, intermuscular septa
Insertion: lateral and dorsal surfaces of second to fifth digits
Nerve: posterior interosseous branch of radial nerve (C7, C8)

Extensor digitorum brevis

Action: extends great toe and adjacent three toes
Origin: superolateral surface of calcaneus, inferior extensor retinaculum, interosseous talocalcaneal ligament
Insertion: base of proximal phalanx of great toe, lateral side of dorsal hood of adjacent three toes
Nerve: deep peroneal nerve (L5, S1)

Extensor digitorum longus

Action: extends lateral four toes, ankle dorsiflexor
Origin: upper three-quarters of medial surface of fibula, interosseous membrane, lateral tibial condyle
Insertion: middle and distal phalanges of four lateral toes
Nerve: deep peroneal nerve (L5, S1)

Extensor hallucis longus

Action: extends great toe, ankle dorsiflexor
Origin: middle half of medial surface of fibula, interosseous membrane
Insertion: base of distal phalanx of great toe
Nerve: deep peroneal nerve (L5)

Extensor indicis

Action: extends index finger and wrist
Origin: lower part of posterior surface of ulna, interosseous membrane
Insertion: dorsal digital expansion on back of proximal phalanx of index finger
Nerve: posterior interosseous nerve (C7, C8)

Extensor pollicis brevis

Action: extends thumb and wrist, abducts wrist
Origin: posterior surface of radius, interosseous membrane
Insertion: dorsolateral base of proximal phalanx of thumb
Nerve: posterior interosseous nerve (C7, C8)

Extensor pollicis longus

Action: extends thumb and wrist, abducts wrist
Origin: middle third of posterior surface of ulna, interosseous membrane
Insertion: dorsal surface of distal phalanx of thumb
Nerve: posterior interosseous nerve (C7, C8)

External oblique

Action: flexes, laterally flexes and rotates trunk
Origin: outer borders of lower eight ribs and their costal cartilages
Insertion: outer lip of anterior two-thirds of iliac crest, abdominal aponeurosis to linea alba stretching from xiphoid process to symphysis pubis
Nerve: ventral rami of lower six thoracic nerves (T7–T12)

Flexor carpi radialis

Action: flexes and abducts wrist
Origin: medial epicondyle via common flexor tendon
Insertion: front of base of second and third metacarpals
Nerve: median (C6, C7)

Flexor carpi ulnaris

Action: flexes and adducts wrist
Origin: humeral head – medial epicondyle via common flexor tendon; ulnar head – medial border of olecranon and upper two-thirds of border of ulna
Insertion: pisiform, hook of hamate and base of fifth metacarpal
Nerve: ulnar nerve (C7–T1)

Flexor digiti minimi brevis (foot)

Action: flexes fifth metatarsophalangeal joint, supports lateral longitudinal arch

Origin: plantar aspect of base of fifth metatarsal, sheath of peroneus longus tendon
Insertion: lateral side of base of proximal phalanx of fifth toe
Nerve: lateral plantar nerve (S2, S3)

Flexor digiti minimi brevis (hand)

Action: flexes little finger
Origin: hook of hamate, flexor retinaculum
Insertion: ulnar side of base of proximal phalanx of little finger
Nerve: ulnar nerve (C8, T1)

Flexor digitorum accessorius

Action: flexes distal phalanges of lateral four toes
Origin: medial head – medial tubercle of calcaneus; lateral head – lateral tubercle of calcaneus and long plantar ligament
Insertion: flexor digitorum longus tendon
Nerve: lateral plantar nerve (S1–S3)

Flexor digitorum brevis

Action: flexes proximal interphalangeal joints and metatarsophalangeal joints of lateral four toes
Origin: calcaneal tuberosity, plantar aponeurosis, intermuscular septa
Insertion: tendons divide and attach to both sides of base of middle phalanges of second to fifth toes
Nerve: medial plantar nerve (S1, S2)

Flexor digitorum longus

Action: flexes lateral four toes, plantarflexes ankle
Origin: medial part of posterior surface of tibia, deep transverse fascia
Insertion: plantar aspect of base of distal phalanges of second to fifth toes
Nerve: tibial nerve (L5–S2)

Flexor digitorum profundus

Action: flexes fingers and wrist
Origin: medial side of coronoid process of ulna, upper three-quarters of anterior and medial surfaces of ulna, interosseous membrane
Insertion: base of palmar surface of distal phalanx of second to fifth digits
Nerve: medial part – ulnar nerve (C8, T1); lateral part – anterior interosseous branch of median nerve (C8, T1)

Flexor digitorum superficialis

Action: flexes fingers and wrist
Origin: humeroulnar head – medial epicondyle via common flexor tendon, medial part of coronoid process of ulna, ulnar collateral ligament, intermuscular septa; radial head – upper two-thirds of anterior border of radius
Insertion: tendons divide and insert into sides of shaft of middle phalanx of second to fifth digits
Nerve: median (C8, T1)

Flexor hallucis brevis

Action: flexes metatarsophalangeal joint of great toe
Origin: medial side of plantar surface of cuboid, lateral cuneiform
Insertion: medial and lateral side of base of proximal phalanx of great toe
Nerve: medial plantar nerve (S1, S2)

Flexor hallucis longus

Action: flexes great toe, plantarflexes ankle
Origin: lower two-thirds of posterior surface of fibula, interosseous membrane, intermuscular septum
Insertion: plantar surface of base of distal phalanx of great toe
Nerve: tibial nerve (L5–S2)

Flexor pollicis brevis

Action: flexes metacarpophalangeal joint of thumb
Origin: flexor retinaculum, tubercle of trapezium, capitate, trapezoid
Insertion: base of proximal phalanx of thumb
Nerve: median nerve (C8–T1). Sometimes also supplied by ulnar nerve (C8–T1)

Flexor pollicis longus

Action: flexes thumb and wrist
Origin: anterior surface of radius, interosseous membrane
Insertion: palmar surface of distal phalanx of thumb
Nerve: anterior interosseous branch of median nerve (C7, C8)

Gastrocnemius

Action: plantarflexes ankle, flexes knee
Origin: medial head – posterior part of medial femoral condyle; lateral head – lateral surface of lateral femoral condyle
Insertion: posterior surface of calcaneus
Nerve: tibial nerve (S1, S2)

Gemellus inferior

Action: laterally rotates hip
Origin: upper part of ischial tuberosity
Insertion: with obturator internus tendon into medial surface of greater trochanter
Nerve: nerve to quadratus femoris (L5, S1)

Gemellus superior

Action: laterally rotates hip
Origin: gluteal surface of ischial spine
Insertion: with obturator internus tendon into medial surface of greater trochanter
Nerve: nerve to obturator internus (L5, S1)

Gluteus maximus

Action: extends, laterally rotates and abducts hip
Origin: posterior gluteal line of ilium, posterior border of ilium and adjacent part of iliac crest, aponeurosis of erector spinae, posterior aspect of sacrum, side of coccyx, sacrotuberous ligament, gluteal aponeurosis
Insertion: iliotibial tract of fascia lata, gluteal tuberosity of femur
Nerve: inferior gluteal nerve (L5–S2)

Gluteus medius

Action: abducts and medially rotates hip
Origin: gluteal surface of ilium between posterior and anterior gluteal lines
Insertion: superolateral side of greater trochanter
Nerve: superior gluteal nerve (L4–S1)

Gluteus minimus

Action: abducts and medially rotates hip
Origin: gluteal surface of ilium between anterior and inferior gluteal lines
Insertion: anterolateral ridge on greater trochanter
Nerve: superior gluteal nerve (L4–S1)

Gracilis

Action: flexes knee, adducts hip, medially rotates tibia on femur
Origin: lower half of body and inferior ramus of pubis, adjacent ischial ramus
Insertion: upper part of medial surface of tibia
Nerve: obturator nerve (L2, L3)

Iliacus

Action: flexes hip and trunk
Origin: superior two-thirds of iliac fossa, inner lip of iliac crest, ala of sacrum, anterior sacroiliac and iliolumbar ligaments

Insertion: blends with insertion of psoas major into lesser trochanter
Nerve: femoral nerve (L2, L3)

Iliocostalis cervicis

Action: extends and laterally flexes vertebral column
Origin: angles of third to sixth ribs
Insertion: posterior tubercles of transverse processes of C4 to C6
Nerve: dorsal rami

Iliocostalis lumborum

Action: extends and laterally flexes vertebral column
Origin: medial and lateral sacral crests, spines of T11, T12 and lumbar vertebrae and their supraspinous ligaments, medial part of iliac crest
Insertion: angles of lower six or seven ribs
Nerve: dorsal rami

Iliocostalis thoracis

Action: extends and laterally flexes vertebral column
Origin: angles of lower six ribs
Insertion: angles of upper six ribs, transverse process of C7
Nerve: dorsal rami

Inferior oblique

Action: rotates atlas and head
Origin: lamina of axis
Insertion: transverse process of atlas
Nerve: dorsal ramus (C1)

Infraspinatus

Action: laterally rotates shoulder
Origin: medial two-thirds of infraspinous fossa and infraspinous fascia

Insertion: middle facet on greater tubercle of humerus, posterior aspect of capsule of shoulder joint
Nerve: suprascapular nerve (C5, C6)

Intercostales externi

Action: elevate rib below towards rib above to increase thoracic cavity volume for inspiration
Origin: lower border of rib above
Insertion: upper border of rib below
Nerve: intercostal nerves

Intercostales interni

Action: draw ribs downwards to decrease thoracic cavity volume for expiration
Origin: lower border of costal cartilage and costal groove of rib above
Insertion: upper border of rib below
Nerve: intercostal nerves

Internal oblique

Action: flexes, laterally flexes and rotates trunk
Origin: lateral two-thirds of inguinal ligament, anterior two-thirds of intermediate line of iliac crest, thoracolumbar fascia
Insertion: lower four ribs and their cartilages, crest of pubis, abdominal aponeurosis to linea alba
Nerve: ventral rami of lower six thoracic nerves, first lumbar nerve

Interspinales

Action: extend and stabilize vertebral column
Origin and insertion: extend between adjacent spinous processes (best developed in cervical and lumbar regions – sometimes absent in thoracic)
Nerve: dorsal rami of spinal nerves

Intertransversarii

Action: laterally flex lumbar and cervical spine, stabilize vertebral column
Origin: transverse processes of cervical and lumbar vertebrae
Insertion: transverse process of vertebra superior to origin
Nerve: ventral and dorsal rami of spinal nerves

Latissimus dorsi

Action: extends, adducts and medially rotates shoulder
Origin: spinous processes of lower six thoracic and all lumbar and sacral vertebrae, intervening supra- and interspinous ligaments, outer lip of iliac crest, outer surfaces of lower three or four ribs, inferior angle of scapula
Insertion: intertubercular sulcus of humerus
Nerve: thoracodorsal nerve (C6–C8)

Levator scapulae

Action: elevates, medially rotates and retracts scapula, extends and laterally flexes neck
Origin: transverse processes of C1–C3/4
Insertion: medial border of scapula between superior angle and base of spine
Nerve: ventral rami (C3, C4), dorsal scapular nerve (C5)

Longissimus capitis

Action: extends, laterally flexes and rotates head
Origin: transverse processes of T1–T4/5, articular processes of C4/5–C7
Insertion: posterior aspect of mastoid process
Nerve: dorsal rami

Longissimus cervicis

Action: extends and laterally flexes vertebral column
Origin: transverse processes of T1–T4/5

Insertion: transverse processes of C2–C6
Nerve: dorsal rami

Longissimus thoracis

Action: extends and laterally flexes vertebral column
Origin: transverse and accessory processes of lumbar vertebrae and thoracolumbar fascia
Insertion: transverse processes of T1–T12 and lower nine or ten ribs
Nerve: dorsal rami

Longus capitis

Action: flexes neck
Origin: occipital bone
Insertion: anterior tubercles of transverse processes of C3–C6
Nerve: anterior primary rami (C1–C3)

Longus colli

Action: flexes neck
Origin: inferior oblique part – front of bodies of T1–T2/3; vertical intermediate part – front of bodies of T1–T3 and C5–C7; superior oblique part – anterior tubercles of transverse processes of C3–C5
Insertion: inferior oblique part – anterior tubercles of transverse processes of C5 and C6; vertical intermediate part – front of bodies of C2–C4; superior oblique part – anterior tubercle of atlas
Nerve: anterior primary rami (C2–C6)

Lumbricals (foot)

Action: flexes metatarsophalangeal joints and extends interphalangeal joints of lateral four toes
Origin: tendons of flexor digitorum longus
Insertion: medial side of extensor hood and base of proximal phalanx of lateral four toes

Nerve: first lumbrical – medial plantar nerve (S2, S3); lateral three lumbricals – lateral plantar nerve (S2, S3)

Lumbricals (hand)

Action: flexes metacarpophalangeal joints and extends interphalangeal joints of fingers
Origin: tendons of flexor digitorum profundus
Insertion: lateral margin of dorsal digital expansion of extensor digitorum
Nerve: first and second – median nerve (C8, T1); third and fourth – ulnar nerve (C8, T1)

Multifidus

Action: extends, rotates and laterally flexes vertebral column
Origin: back of sacrum, aponeurosis of erector spinae, posterior superior iliac spine, dorsal sacroiliac ligaments, mamillary processes in lumbar region, all thoracic transverse processes, articular processes of lower four cervical vertebrae
Insertion: spines of all vertebrae from L5 to axis (deep layer attaches to vertebrae above; middle layer attaches to second or third vertebrae above; outer layer attaches to third or fourth vertebrae above)
Nerve: dorsal rami of spinal nerves

Obturator externus

Action: laterally rotates hip
Origin: outer surface of obturator membrane and adjacent bone of pubic and ischial rami
Insertion: trochanteric fossa of femur
Nerve: posterior branch of obturator nerve (L3, L4)

Obturator internus

Action: laterally rotates hip
Origin: internal surface of obturator membrane and surrounding bony margin

Insertion: medial surface of greater trochanter
Nerve: nerve to obturator internus (L5, S1)

Opponens digiti minimi

Action: abducts fifth digit, pulls it forwards and rotates it laterally
Origin: hook of hamate, flexor retinaculum
Insertion: medial border of fifth metacarpal
Nerve: ulnar nerve (C8, T1)

Opponens pollicis

Action: rotates thumb into opposition with fingers
Origin: flexor retinaculum, tubercles of scaphoid and trapezium, abductor pollicis longus tendon
Insertion: radial side of base of proximal phalanx of thumb
Nerve: median nerve (C8, T1)

Palmar interossei

Action: adducts thumb, index, ring and little finger
Origin: shaft of metacarpal of digit on which it acts
Insertion: dorsal digital expansion and base of proximal phalanx of same digit
Nerve: ulnar nerve (C8, T1)

Palmaris longus

Action: flexes wrist
Origin: medial epicondyle via common flexor tendon
Insertion: flexor retinaculum, palmar aponeurosis
Nerve: median (C7, C8)

Pectineus

Action: flexes and adducts hip
Origin: pecten pubis, iliopectineal eminence, pubic tubercle

Insertion: along a line from lesser trochanter to linea aspera
Nerve: femoral nerve (L2, L3), occasionally accessory obturator (L3)

Pectoralis major

Action: adducts, medially rotates, flexes and extends shoulder
Origin: clavicular attachment – sternal half of anterior surface of clavicle; sternocostal attachment – anterior surface of manubrium, body of sternum, upper six costal cartilages, sixth rib, aponeurosis of external oblique muscle
Insertion: lateral lip of intertubercular sulcus of humerus
Nerve: medial and lateral pectoral nerves (C5–T1)

Pectoralis minor

Action: protracts and medially rotates scapula
Origin: outer surface of third to fifth ribs and adjoining intercostal fascia
Insertion: upper surface and medial border of coracoid process
Nerve: medial and lateral pectoral nerves (C5–T1)

Peroneus brevis

Action: everts and plantarflexes ankle
Origin: lower two-thirds of lateral surface of fibula, intermuscular septa
Insertion: lateral side of base of fifth metatarsal
Nerve: superficial peroneal nerve (L5, S1)

Peroneus longus

Action: everts and plantarflexes ankle
Origin: lateral tibial condyle, upper two-thirds of lateral surface of fibula, intermuscular septa
Insertion: lateral side of base of first metatarsal, medial cuneiform
Nerve: superficial peroneal nerve (L5, S1)

Peroneus tertius

Action: everts and dorsiflexes ankle
Origin: distal third of medial surface of fibula, interosseous membrane, intermuscular septum
Insertion: medial aspect of base of fifth metatarsal
Nerve: deep peroneal nerve (L5, S1)

Piriformis

Action: laterally rotates and abducts hip
Origin: front of second to fourth sacral segments, gluteal surface of ilium, pelvic surface of sacrotuberous ligament
Insertion: medial side of greater trochanter
Nerve: anterior rami of sacral plexus (L5–S2)

Plantar interossei

Action: adduct third to fifth toes, flex metatarsophalangeal joints of lateral three toes
Origin: base and medial side of lateral three toes
Insertion: medial side of base of proximal phalanx of same toes and dorsal digital expansions
Nerve: lateral plantar nerve (S2, S3)

Plantaris

Action: plantarflexes ankle, flexes knee
Origin: lateral supracondylar ridge, oblique popliteal ligament
Insertion: tendocalcaneus
Nerve: tibial nerve (S1, S2)

Popliteus

Action: medially rotates tibia, flexes knee
Origin: outer surface of lateral femoral condyle
Insertion: posterior surface of tibia above soleal line
Nerve: tibial nerve (L4–S1)

Pronator quadratus

Action: pronates forearm
Origin: lower quarter of anterior surface of ulna
Insertion: lower quarter of anterior surface of radius
Nerve: anterior interosseous branch of median nerve (C7, C8)

Pronator teres

Action: pronates forearm, flexes elbow
Origin: humeral head – medial epicondyle via common flexor tendon, intermuscular septum, antebrachial fascia; ulnar head – medial part of coronoid process
Insertion: middle of lateral surface of radius
Nerve: median nerve (C6, C7)

Psoas major

Action: flexes hip and lumbar spine
Origin: bodies of T12 and all lumbar vertebrae, bases of transverse processes of all lumbar vertebrae, lumbar intervertebral discs
Insertion: lesser trochanter
Nerve: anterior rami of lumbar plexus (L1–L3)

Psoas minor (not always present)

Action: flexes trunk (weak)
Origin: bodies of T12 and L1 vertebrae and intervertebral discs
Insertion: pecten pubis, iliopubic eminence, iliac fascia
Nerve: anterior primary ramus (L1)

Quadratus femoris

Action: laterally rotates hip
Origin: ischial tuberosity

Insertion: quadrate tubercle midway down intertrochanteric crest
Nerve: nerve to quadratus femoris (L5, S1)

Quadratus lumborum

Action: laterally flexes trunk, extends lumbar vertebrae, steadies twelfth rib during deep inspiration
Origin: iliolumbar ligament, posterior part of iliac crest
Insertion: lower border of twelfth rib, transverse processes of L1–L4
Nerve: ventral rami of T12 and L1–L3/4

Rectus abdominis

Action: flexes trunk
Origin: symphysis pubis, pubic crest
Insertion: fifth to seventh costal cartilages, xiphoid process
Nerve: ventral rami of T6/7–T12

Rectus capitis anterior

Action: flexes neck
Origin: anterior surface of lateral mass of atlas and root of its transverse process
Insertion: occipital bone
Nerve: anterior primary rami (C1, C2)

Rectus capitis lateralis

Action: laterally flexes neck
Origin: transverse process of atlas
Insertion: jugular process of occipital bone
Nerve: ventral rami (C1, C2)

Rectus capitis posterior major

Action: extends and rotates neck

Origin: spinous process of axis
Insertion: lateral part of inferior nuchal line of occipital bone
Nerve: dorsal ramus (C1)

Rectus capitis posterior minor

Action: extends neck
Origin: posterior tubercle of atlas
Insertion: medial part of inferior nuchal line of occipital bone
Nerve: dorsal ramus (C1)

Rectus femoris

Action: extends knee, flexes hip
Origin: straight head – anterior inferior iliac spine; reflected head – area above acetabulum, capsule of hip joint
Insertion: base of patella, then forms part of patellar ligament
Nerve: femoral nerve (L2–L4)

Rhomboid major

Action: retracts and medially rotates scapula
Origin: spines and supraspinous ligaments of T2–T5
Insertion: medial border of scapula between root of spine and inferior angle
Nerve: dorsal scapular nerve (C4, C5)

Rhomboid minor

Action: retracts and medially rotates scapula
Origin: spines and supraspinous ligaments of C7–T1, lower part of ligamentum nuchae
Insertion: medial end of spine of scapula
Nerve: dorsal scapular nerve (C4, C5)

Rotatores

Action: extends vertebral column and rotates thoracic region
Origin: transverse process of each vertebra
Insertion: lamina of vertebra above
Nerve: dorsal rami of spinal nerves

Sartorius

Action: flexes hip and knee, laterally rotates and abducts hip, medially rotates tibia on femur
Origin: anterior superior iliac spine and area just below
Insertion: upper part of medial side of tibia
Nerve: femoral nerve (L2, L3)

Scalenus anterior

Action: flexes, laterally flexes and rotates neck, raises first rib during respiration
Origin: anterior tubercles of transverse processes of C3–C6
Insertion: scalene tubercle on inner border of first rib
Nerve: ventral rami (C4–C6)

Scalenus medius

Action: laterally flexes neck, raises first rib during respiration
Origin: transverse processes of atlas and axis, posterior tubercles of transverse processes of C3–C7
Insertion: upper surface of first rib
Nerve: ventral rami (C3–C8)

Scalenus posterior

Action: laterally flexes neck, raises second rib during respiration
Origin: posterior tubercles of transverse processes of C4–C6
Insertion: outer surface of second rib
Nerve: ventral rami (C6–C8)

Semimembranosus

Action: flexes knee, extends hip and medially rotates tibia on femur
Origin: ischial tuberosity
Insertion: posterior aspect of medial tibial condyle
Nerve: tibial division of sciatic nerve (L5–S2)

Semispinalis capitis

Action: extends and rotates head
Origin: transverse processes of C7–T6/7, articular processes of C4–C6
Insertion: between superior and inferior nuchal lines of occipital bone
Nerve: dorsal rami of spinal nerves

Semispinalis cervicis

Action: extends and rotates vertebral column
Origin: transverse processes of T1–T5/6
Insertion: spinous processes of C2–C5
Nerve: dorsal rami of spinal nerves

Semispinalis thoracis

Action: extends and rotates vertebral column
Origin: transverse processes of T6–T10
Insertion: spinous processes of C6–T4
Nerve: dorsal rami of spinal nerves

Semitendinosus

Action: flexes knee, extends hip and medially rotates tibia on femur
Origin: ischial tuberosity
Insertion: upper part of medial surface of tibia
Nerve: tibial division of sciatic nerve (L5–S2)

Serratus anterior

Action: protracts and laterally rotates scapula
Origin: outer surfaces and superior borders of upper eight, nine or ten ribs and intervening intercostal fascia
Insertion: costal surface of medial border of scapula
Nerve: long thoracic nerve (C5–C7)

Soleus

Action: plantarflexes ankle
Origin: soleal line and middle third of medial border of tibia, posterior surface of head and upper quarter of fibula, fibrous arch between tibia and fibula
Insertion: posterior surface of calcaneus
Nerve: tibial nerve (S1, S2)

Spinalis (capitis*, cervicis*, thoracis)

Action: extends vertebral column
Origin: spinalis thoracis – spinous processes of T11–L2
Insertion: spinalis thoracis – spinous processes of upper four to eight thoracic vertebrae
* Spinalis capitis and spinalis cervicis are poorly developed and blend with adjacent muscles
Nerve: dorsal rami

Splenius capitis

Action: extends, laterally flexes and rotates neck
Origin: lower half of ligamentum nuchae, spinous processes of C7–T3/4 and their supraspinous ligaments
Insertion: mastoid process of temporal bone, lateral third of superior nuchal line of occipital bone
Nerve: dorsal rami (C3–C5)

Splenius cervicis

Action: laterally flexes, rotates and extends neck

Origin: spinous processes of T3–T6
Insertion: posterior tubercles of transverse processes of C1–C3/4
Nerve: dorsal rami (C5–C7)

Sternocleidomastoid

Action: laterally flexes and rotates neck; anterior fibres flex neck, posterior fibres extend neck
Origin: sternal head – anterior surface of manubrium sterni; clavicular head – upper surface of medial third of clavicle
Insertion: mastoid process of temporal bone, lateral half of superior nuchal line of occipital bone
Nerve: accessory nerve (XI)

Subscapularis

Action: medially rotates shoulder
Origin: medial two-thirds of subscapular fossa and tendinous intramuscular septa
Insertion: lesser tubercle of humerus, anterior capsule of shoulder joint
Nerve: upper and lower subscapular nerves (C5, C6)

Superior oblique

Action: extends neck
Origin: upper surface of transverse process of atlas
Insertion: superior and inferior nuchal lines of occipital bone
Nerve: dorsal ramus (C1)

Supinator

Action: supinates forearm
Origin: inferior aspect of lateral epicondyle, radial collateral ligament, annular ligament, supinator crest and fossa of ulna
Insertion: posterior, lateral and anterior aspects of upper third of radius
Nerve: posterior interosseous nerve (C6, C7)

Supraspinatus

Action: abducts shoulder
Origin: medial two-thirds of supraspinous fossa and supraspinous fascia
Insertion: capsule of shoulder joint, greater tubercle of humerus
Nerve: suprascapular nerve (C5, C6)

Tensor fascia lata

Action: extends knee, abducts and medially rotates hip
Origin: outer lip of iliac crest between iliac tubercle and anterior superior iliac spine
Insertion: iliotibial tract
Nerve: superior gluteal nerve (L4–S1)

Teres major

Action: extends, adducts and medially rotates shoulder
Origin: dorsal surface of inferior scapular angle
Insertion: medial lip of intertubercular sulcus of humerus
Nerve: lower subscapular nerve (C5–C7)

Teres minor

Action: laterally rotates shoulder
Origin: upper two-thirds of dorsal surface of scapula
Insertion: lower facet on greater tuberosity of humerus, lower posterior surface of capsule of shoulder joint
Nerve: axillary nerve (C5, C6)

Tibialis anterior

Action: dorsiflexes and inverts ankle
Origin: lateral tibial condyle and upper two-thirds of lateral surface of tibia, interosseous membrane
Insertion: medial and inferior surface of medial cuneiform, base of first metatarsal
Nerve: deep peroneal nerve (L4, L5)

Tibialis posterior

Action: plantarflexes and inverts ankle
Origin: lateral aspect of posterior surface of tibia below soleal line, interosseous membrane, upper half of posterior surface of fibula, deep transverse fascia
Insertion: tuberosity of navicular, medial cuneiform, sustentaculum tali, intermediate cuneiform, base of second to fourth metatarsals
Nerve: tibial nerve (L4, L5)

Transversus abdominis

Action: compresses abdominal contents, raises intra-abdominal pressure
Origin: lateral third of inguinal ligament, anterior two-thirds of inner lip of iliac crest, thoracolumbar fascia between iliac crest and twelfth rib, lower six costal cartilages where it interdigitates with diaphragm
Insertion: abdominal aponeurosis to linea alba
Nerve: ventral rami of lower six thoracic and first lumbar spinal nerve

Trapezius

Action: upper fibres elevate scapula, middle fibres retract scapula, lower fibres depress scapula, upper and lower fibres together laterally rotate scapula. Also extends and laterally flexes head and neck
Origin: medial third of superior nuchal line, external occipital protuberance, ligamentum nuchae, spinous processes and supraspinous ligaments of C7–T12
Insertion: upper fibres – posterior border of lateral third of clavicle; middle fibres – medial border of acromion, superior lip of crest of spine of scapula; lower fibres – tubercle at medial end of spine of scapula
Nerve: accessory nerve (XI), ventral rami (C3, C4)

Triceps brachii

Action: extends elbow and shoulder
Origin: long head – infraglenoid tubercle of scapula, shoulder capsule; lateral head – above and lateral to spiral groove on posterior surface of humerus; medial head – below and medial to spiral groove on posterior surface of humerus
Insertion: upper surface of olecranon, deep fascia of forearm
Nerve: radial nerve (C6–C8)

Vastus intermedius

Action: extends knee
Origin: upper two-thirds of anterior and lateral surfaces of femur, lower part of lateral intermuscular septum
Insertion: deep surface of quadriceps tendon, lateral border of patella, lateral tibial condyle
Nerve: femoral nerve (L2–L4)

Vastus lateralis

Action: extends knee
Origin: intertrochanteric line, greater trochanter, gluteal tuberosity, lateral lip of linea aspera
Insertion: tendon of rectus femoris, lateral border of patella
Nerve: femoral nerve (L2–L4)

Vastus medialis

Action: extends knee
Origin: intertrochanteric line, spiral line, medial lip of linea aspera, medial supracondylar line, medial intermuscular septum, tendons of adductor longus and adductor magnus
Insertion: tendon of rectus femoris, medial border of patella, medial tibial condyle
Nerve: femoral nerve (L2–L4)

Common postures (from Kendall et al 1993, with permission of Lippincott Williams & Wilkins)

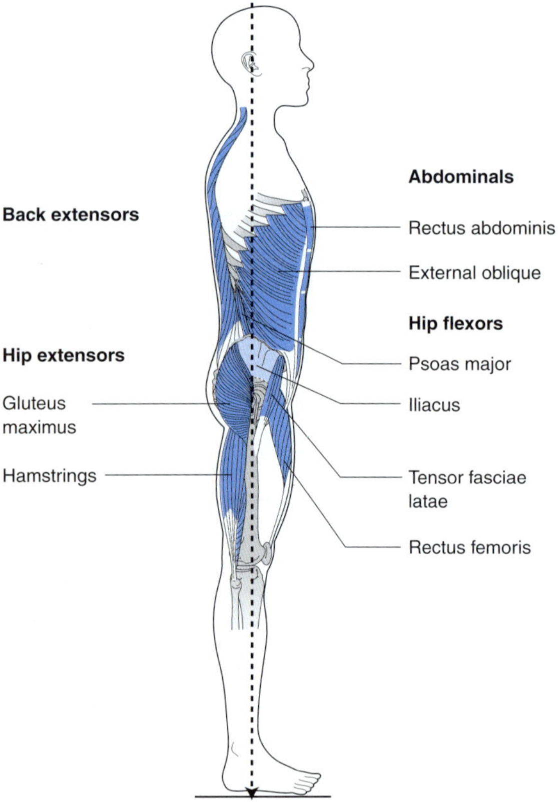

Figure 1.19 Ideal alignment (side view).

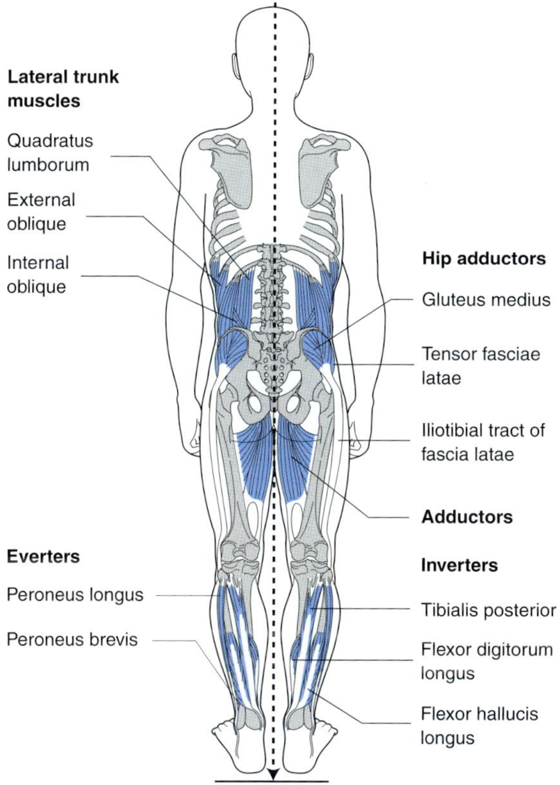

Figure 1.20 Ideal alignment (posterior view).

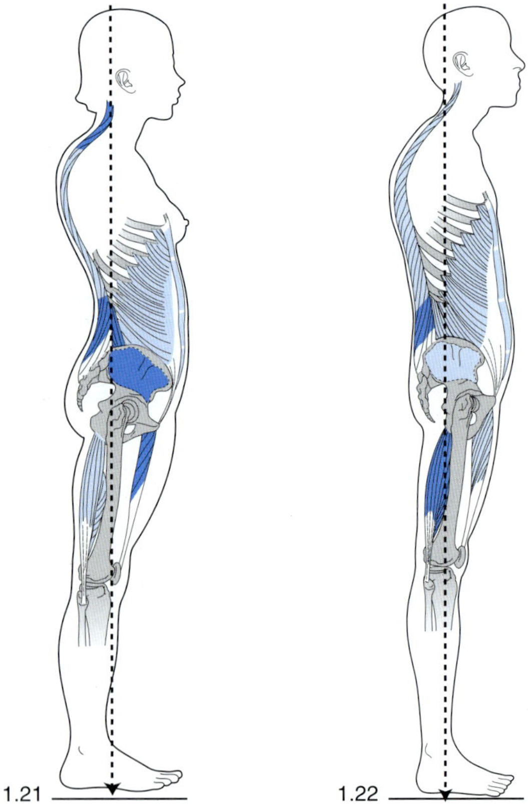

Figure 1.21 Kyphosis – lordosis posture.

Figure 1.22 Sway-back posture.

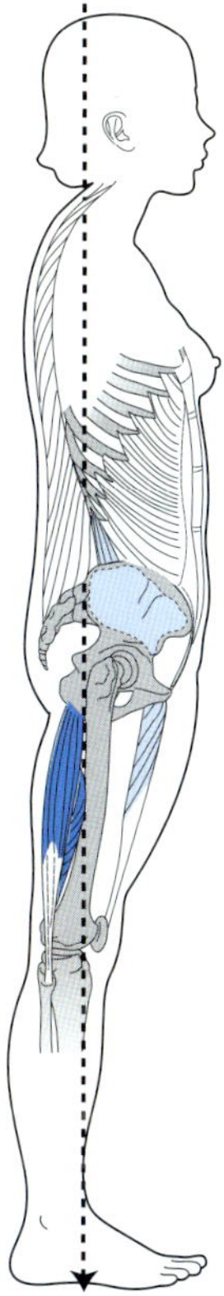
1.23

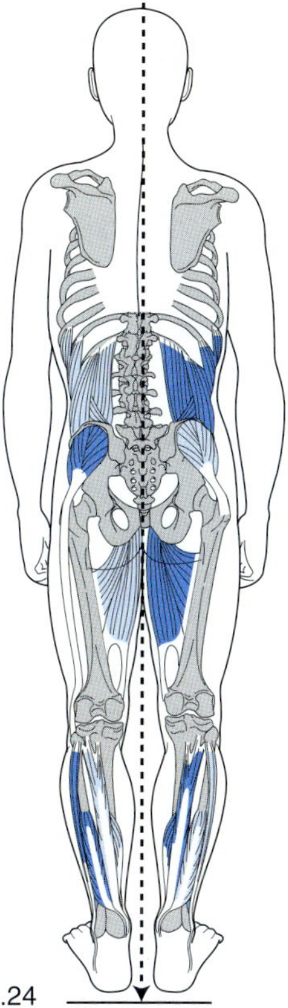
1.24

Figure 1.23 Flat-back posture.

Figure 1.24 Faulty alignment (posterior view). Typical of right-handed individuals.

Ideal alignment: side view (Fig. 1.19)

Anteriorly, the abdominal muscles pull upward and the hip flexors pull downward. Posteriorly, the back muscles pull upward and the hip extensors pull downward. Thus, the abdominal and hip extensor muscles work together to tilt the pelvis posteriorly; the back and hip flexor muscles work together to tilt the pelvis anteriorly.

Ideal alignment: posterior view (Fig. 1.20)

Laterally, the following groups of muscles work together in stabilizing the trunk, pelvis and lower extremities:

- Right lateral trunk flexors
- Right hip adductors
- Left hip abductors
- Right tibialis posterior
- Right flexor hallucis longus
- Right flexor digitorum longus
- Left peroneus longus and brevis

- Left lateral trunk flexors
- Left hip adductors
- Right hip abductors
- Left tibialis posterior
- Left flexor hallucis longus
- Left flexor digitorum longus
- Right peroneus longus and brevis

Kyphosis–lordosis posture (Fig. 1.21)

Short and strong: neck extensors and hip flexors. The low back is strong and may or may not develop shortness.

Elongated and weak: neck flexors, upper back erector spinae and external oblique. Hamstrings are slightly elongated but may or may not be weak.

Sway-back posture (Fig. 1.22)

Short and strong: hamstrings and upper fibres of internal oblique. *Strong but not short*: lumbar erector spinae.

Elongated and weak: one-joint hip flexors, external oblique, upper back extensors and neck flexors.

Flat-back posture (Fig. 1.23)

Short and strong: hamstrings and often the abdominals.
Elongated and weak: one-joint hip flexors.

Faulty alignment: posterior view (Fig. 1.24)

Short and strong: right lateral trunk muscles, left hip abductors, right hip adductors, left peroneus longus and brevis, right tibialis posterior, right flexor hallucis longus, right flexor digitorum longus. The left tensor fascia lata is usually strong and there may be tightness in the iliotibial band.

Elongated and weak: left lateral trunk muscles, right hip abductors (especially posterior gluteus medius), left hip adductors, right peroneus longus and brevis, left tibialis posterior, left flexor hallucis longus, left flexor digitorum longus. The right tensor fascia lata may or may not be weak.

Joint range of movement (from McRae 1999, with permission)

Cervical spine

Flexion	0–80°
Extension	0–50°
Total flexion/extension	0–130°
Lateral side flexion	0–45°
Rotation to each side	0–80°

Shoulder

Flexion	0–165°
Extension	0–60°
Abduction	0–170°
Internal rotation at 90° abduction	0–70°
External rotation at 90° abduction	0–100°

Elbow

Flexion	0–145°
Extension	0°
Pronation	0–75°
Supination	0–80°

Wrist

Flexion	0–75°
Extension	0–75°
Radial deviation	0–20°
Ulnar deviation	0–35°
Pronation	0–75°
Supination	0–80°

Thumb

IP joint flexion	0–80°
IP joint extension	0–20°
MP joint flexion	0–55°
MP joint extension, passive	0–5°
Carpo-metacarpal abduction	0–20°
Carpo-metacarpal flexion	0–15°

Fingers

MP joints, flexion	0–90°
MP joints, passive hyperextension	up to 45°
Proximal IP joints, flexion	0–100°
Distal IP joints, flexion	0–80°

Thoracolumbar spine

Thoracic spine flexion	0–45°
Lumbar spine flexion	0–60°
Combined lateral flexion to each side	0–30°
Thoracic spine rotation to each side	0–40°

Hip

Flexion	0–120°
Extension	5–20°
Abduction	0–40°
Adduction	0 25°
Internal rotation at 90° flexion	0–45°
External rotation at 90° flexion	0–45°
Internal rotation in extension	0–35°
External rotation in extension	0–45°

Knee

Flexion	0–135°+
Extension	0°

Ankle

Dorsiflexion	0–15°
Plantarflexion	0–55°

Foot

Inversion of heel	0–20°
Eversion of heel	0–10°
Total supination at forefoot level	0–35°
Total pronation at forefoot level	0–20°

Great toe

Flexion at MP joint	0–40°
Extension at MP joint	0–65°
Flexion at IP joint	0–60°
Extension at IP joint	0°

Note

MP, metatarsophalangeal/metacarpophalangeal joints; IP, interphalangeal joints.

Close packed positions and capsular patterns for selected joints

Joint	Close packed position	Capsular pattern*
Temporomandibular	Clenched teeth	Opening mouth
Cervical spine	Extension (also applies to thoracic and lumbar spine)	Side flexion and rotation equally limited; flexion is full but painful, extension is limited
Glenohumeral	Abduction and lateral rotation	Lateral rotation then abduction then medial rotation
Humeroulnar	Extension	Flexion then extension
Radiocarpal	Extension with radial deviation	Flexion and extension equally limited
Trapeziometacarpal	None	Abduction and extension, full flexion
Metacarpophalangeal and interphalangeal	*Metacarpophalangeal* Flexion (fingers) Opposition (thumb) *Interphalangeal* Extension	Flexion then extension

Hip	Extension and medial rotation	Flexion, abduction and medial rotation (order may vary) Extension is slightly limited
Knee	Extension and lateral rotation of tibia	Flexion then extension
Talocrural	Dorsiflexion	Plantarflexion then dorsiflexion
Subtalar	Inversion	Inversion
Mid-tarsal	Inversion (also applies to tarsometatarsal)	Dorsiflexion, plantarflexion, adduction and medial rotation
First metatarsophalangeal	*Metatarsophalangeal* Extension *Interphalangeal* Extension	Extension then flexion

*Movements are listed in order of restriction, from the most limited to the least limited.
Data from Cyriax (1982) and Magee (2002).

Peripheral nerve pathways (Figs 1.25–1.31 from O'Brian 2000, with permission)

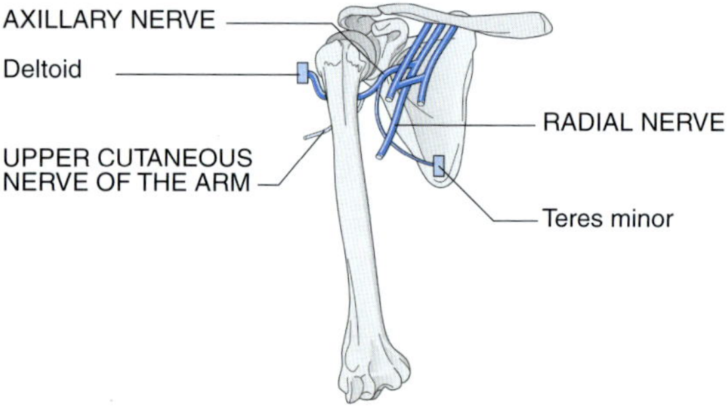

Figure 1.25 Upper cutaneous nerve of the arm.

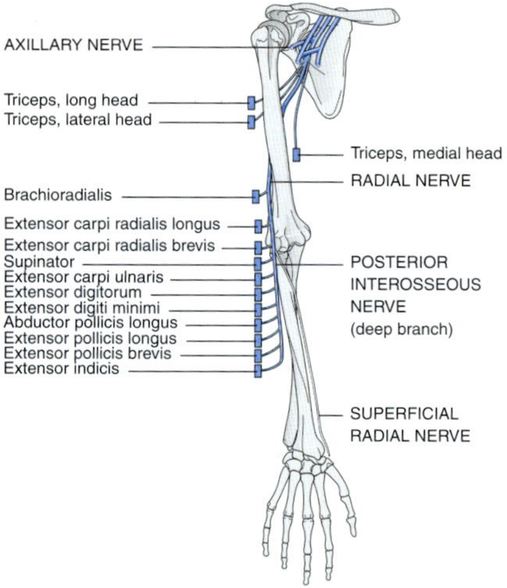

Figure 1.26 Axillary and radial nerve.

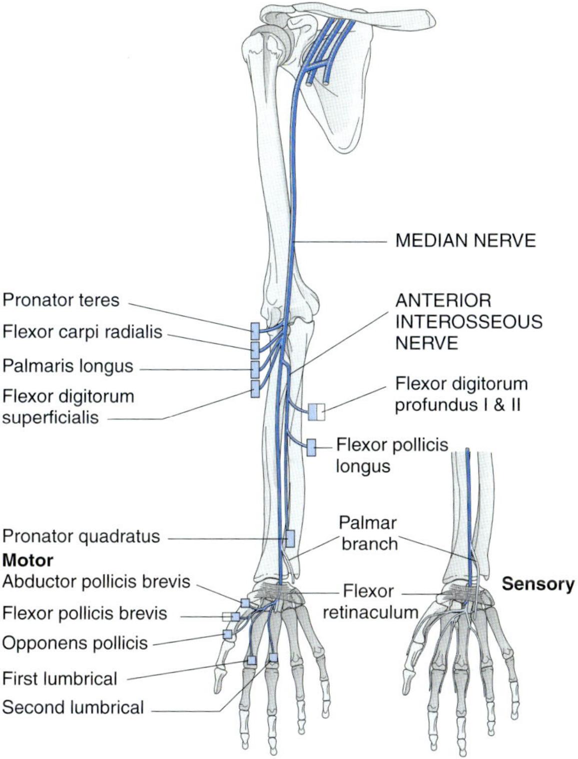

Figure 1.27 Median nerve.

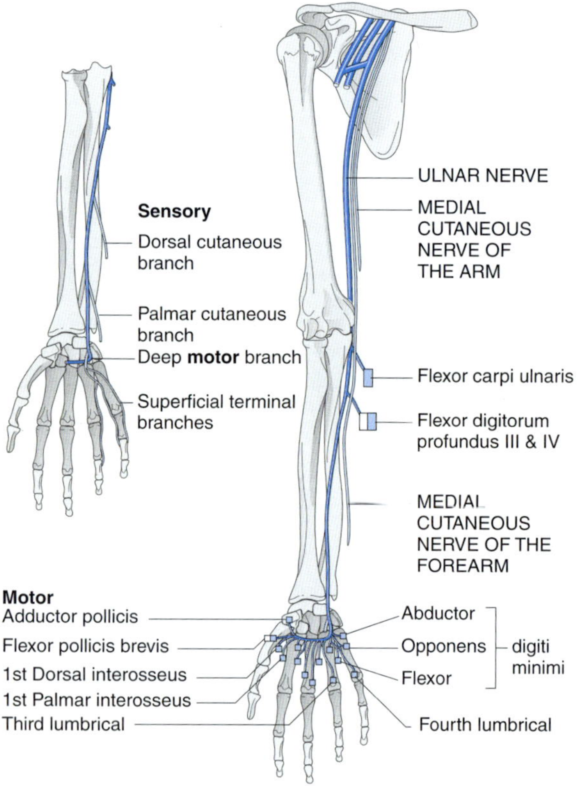

Figure 1.28 Ulnar nerve.

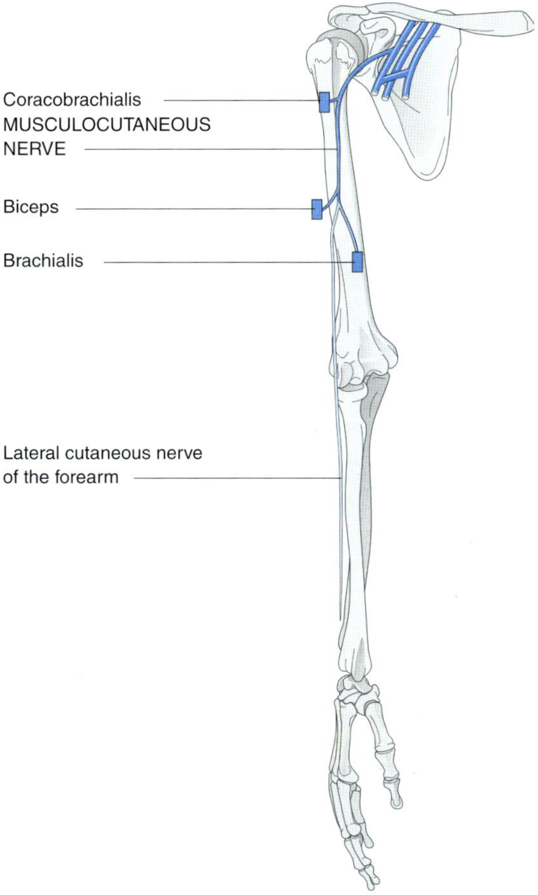

Figure 1.29 Musculocutaneous nerve.

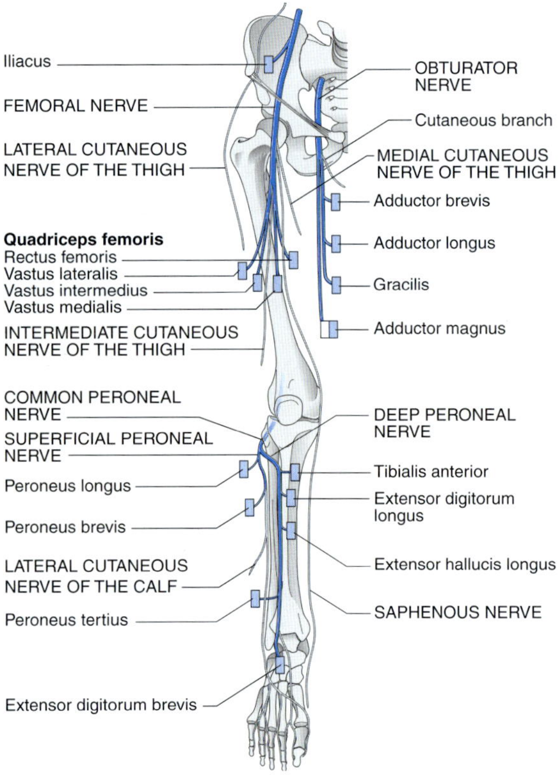

Figure 1.30 Anterior aspect of lower limb.

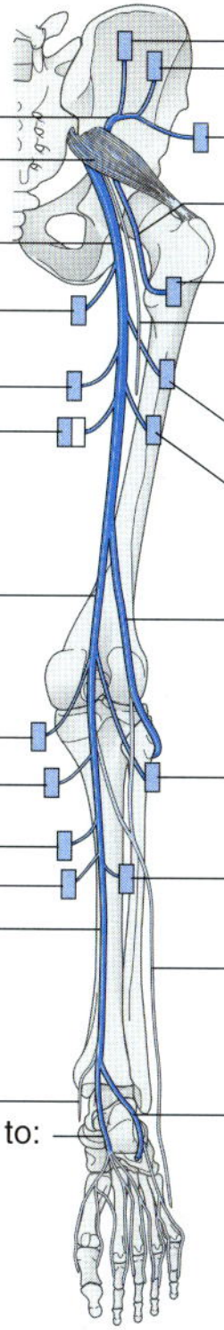

Figure 1.31 Posterior aspect of lower limb.

Dermatomes (from O'Brian 2000, with permission)

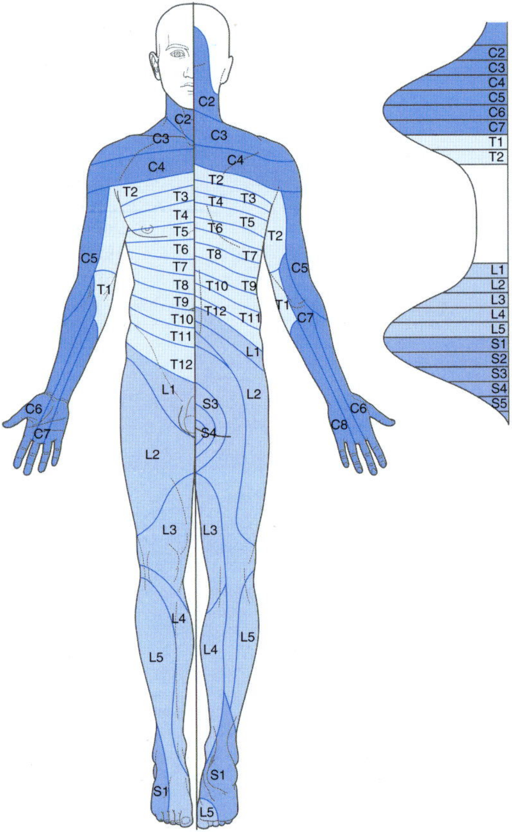

Figure 1.32 Dermatomes of the whole body.

Myotomes (adapted from Grieve 1991, with permission)

Root	Joint action	Root	Joint action
C1	Upper cervical flexion	T1	Finger abduction/ adduction
C2	Upper cervical extension	T2–L1	No muscle test
		L2	Hip flexion
C3	Cervical lateral flexion	L3	Knee extension
		L4	Dorsiflexion
C4	Shoulder girdle elevation	L5	Great toe extension
C5	Shoulder abduction	S1	Eversion
C6	Elbow flexion		Contract buttock
C7	Elbow extension		Knee flexion
C8	Thumb extension; finger flexion	S2	Knee flexion Toe standing

Reflexes

Deep tendon reflex	Root	Nerve
Biceps jerk	C5–C6	Musculocutaneous
Brachioradialis jerk	C5–C6	Radial
Triceps jerk	C7–C8	Radial
Knee jerk	L3–L4	Femoral
Ankle jerk	S1–S2	Tibial

Pathological reflex	Positive response	Pathology
Babinski	Extension of big toe and fanning of other toes in response to scraping stimulus up the lateral border of the sole of the foot and across the foot pad	Upper motor neurone lesion
Clonus	More than three rhythmic contractions of the plantar-flexors in response to sudden passive dorsiflexion	Upper motor neurone lesion

Common locations for palpation of pulses

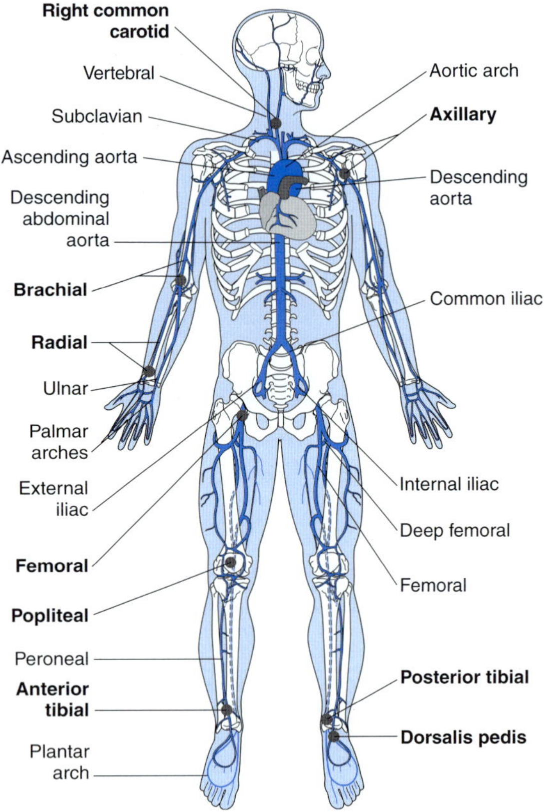

Figure 1.33 Pulse points.

Common carotid	Between the trachea and the sternocleidomastoid muscle
Axillary	Lateral wall of axilla in the groove behind coracobrachialis
Brachial	a) Between the humerus and biceps on the medial aspect of arm b) Cubital fossa
Radial	Lateral to flexor carpi radialis tendon
Femoral	In femoral triangle (sartorius, adductor longus and inguinal ligament)
Popliteal	In popliteal fossa. Palpated more easily in prone with the knee flexed about 45°
Anterior tibial	Above level of ankle joint, between tibialis anterior and extensor hallucis longus tendons
Posterior tibial	Posterior aspect of medial malleolus
Dorsalis pedis	Dorsum of foot, between first and second metatarsal bones

Musculoskeletal pathologies

Ankylosing spondylitis

A chronic inflammatory disease of synovial joints, involving the joint capsule and its attached ligaments and tendons. The spinal and sacroiliac joints are primarily affected resulting in pain, stiffness, fatigue, loss of movement and function. As the disease progresses the vertebrae fuse together. The disease is more common in young males.

Baker's cyst

Distension of the popliteal bursa, which may be accompanied by herniation of the synovial membrane of the knee-joint capsule forming a fluid-filled sac at the back of the knee. Associated with rheumatoid arthritis and osteoarthritis.

Bursitis

Inflammation of the bursa caused by mechanical irritation or infection. Bursas that are commonly affected include the prepatellar, olecranon (can be associated with gout), subacromial, trochanteric, semimembranosus and the 'bunion' associated with hallux valgus. May or may not be painful.

Carpal tunnel syndrome

Compression of the median nerve as it passes beneath the flexor retinaculum, caused by inflammation due to joint disease, trauma, repetitive injury or during menopause. Characterized by pain, numbness, tingling or burning sensation in the distribution of the median nerve, i.e. the radial three and a half fingers and nail beds and the associated area of the palm. Symptoms are often worse at night. Patients also complain of clumsiness performing fine movements of the hand, particularly in the early morning.

Compartment syndrome

Soft tissue ischaemia caused by increased pressure in a fascial compartment of a limb. This increased pressure can have a number of causes but the main ones are swelling following major trauma, a cast being applied too tightly over an injured limb, or repetitive strain injury. Signs and symptoms are pain, pale/plum colour, absent pulse, paraesthesia and loss of active movement. If left untreated, it leads to necrosis of nerve and muscle in the affected compartment, which is known as Volkmann's ischaemic contracture.

Complex regional pain syndrome (CRPS)

An umbrella term for a number of conditions, usually affecting the distal extremities, whose common features include unremitting severe pain (often described as burning) and autonomic changes in the affected region such as swelling, tenderness, restriction of movement, increased skin temperature, sweating, discoloration of the skin (usually blue or dusky red) and osteoporosis. CRPS is subdivided into two groups:

Group II – conditions where there has been an injury to a major peripheral nerve (e.g. sciatic nerve). Also referred to as causalgia ('hot pain').

Group I – conditions where minor or major trauma has occurred but there is no identifiable nerve injury, e.g. after Colles' fractures. Also referred to as reflex sympathetic dystrophy and Sudeck's atrophy.

Dupuytren's contracture

Thickening and shortening of the palmar aponeurosis together with flexion contracture of one or more fingers. The cause is unknown.

Fibromyalgia/fibrositis

A non-articular rheumatological disorder associated with widespread myofascial and joint pain and pain and tenderness in at least 11 of 18 trigger points. Other problems associated with fibromyalgia include fatigue, disturbed sleep, depression, anxiety and morning stiffness. The cause and pathogenesis of fibromyalgia is unknown, but it can either develop on its own or together with other conditions such as rheumatoid arthritis or systemic lupus erythematosus.

Ganglion

An abnormal but harmless cystic swelling that often develops over a tendon sheath or joint capsule, especially on the back of the wrist.

Golfer's elbow (medial epicondylitis)

Tendinopathy of the common origin of the forearm flexors causing pain and tenderness at the medial aspect of the elbow and down the forearm.

Myositis ossificans

Growth of bone in the soft tissues near a joint that occurs after fracture or severe soft tissue trauma, particularly around the elbow. Also occurs in a congenital progressive form, usually leading to early death during adolescence.

Osteoarthritis

A chronic disease of articular cartilage, associated with secondary changes in the underlying bone, causing joint inflammation and degeneration. Primarily affects the large, weight-bearing joints such as the knee and hip, resulting in pain, loss of movement and loss of normal function.

Osteochrondritis

An umbrella term for a variety of conditions where there is compression, fragmentation or separation of a piece of bone.

Perthes' disease

Seen mainly in young boys, it affects the upper femoral epiphysis, which becomes ischaemic and necrotic. The tissues of the femoral head become soft and fragmented but eventually reform over a period of several years. However, the reformed head is flatter and larger than the original, which can lead to deformity, shortening and secondary osteoarthritis. The cause is unknown.

Osgood–Schlatter's disease

Seen mainly in teenage boys, it affects the tibial tubercle. Vigorous physical activity can cause the patellar tendon to pull at its attachment to the tibial tuberosity resulting in detachment of small cartilage fragments.

Osteochrondritis dissecans

Seen mainly in adolescent boys, it is a gradual localized separation of a fragment of bone and cartilage into a joint. The medial femoral condyle and the capitulum of the humerus are the most common sites. The loose body can enter the joint space resulting in pain, swelling and reduced movement.

Scheuermann's disease

Seen mainly in adolescent boys, it is a growth disturbance of the thoracic vertebral bodies, resulting in degeneration of the intervertebral disc into the vertebral endplate. Can lead to a thoracic kyphosis of varying severity.

Osteomalacia

Softening of the bone caused by a deficiency in vitamin D from poor nutrition, lack of sunshine or problems absorbing or metabolizing vitamin D. A lack of vitamin D leads to incomplete calcification of the bones so that they become weak and easily fractured. This is particularly noticeable in the long bones, which become bowed. In children, the condition is called rickets.

Osteomyelitis

An inflammation of the bone and bone marrow due to infection. The most common causes are infection of an open fracture or postoperatively after bone or joint surgery. The infection is often spread from another part of the body to the bone via the blood.

Osteoporosis

A reduction in bone density which results from the body being unable to form enough new bone or when too much calcium and phosphate is reabsorbed back into the body from existing bones. This leads to thin, weak, brittle bones that are susceptible to fracture. Osteoporosis is common in post-menopausal women where a loss of ovarian function results in a reduction in oestrogen production. It can also be caused by prolonged disuse and non-weight bearing, endocrine disorders such as Cushing's disease, and steroid therapy.

Paget's disease

Characterized by an excessive amount of bone breakdown associated with abnormal bone formation causing the bones to become enlarged, deformed and weak. Normal architecture of the trabeculae is affected making the bones brittle. Paget's disease is usually confined to individual bones although more than one bone can be affected. Also known as osteitis deformans. The cause remains unknown.

Polyarteritis nodosa

A vasculitic syndrome where small and medium-sized arteries are attacked by rogue immune cells causing inflammation and necrosis. Tissue supplied by the affected arteries, most commonly the skin, heart, kidneys and nervous system, is damaged by the impaired blood supply. Common manifestations are fever, renal failure, hypertension, neuritis, skin lesions, weight loss and muscle and joint pain.

Polymyalgia rheumatica

A vasculitic syndrome associated with fever and generalized pain and stiffness, especially in the shoulder and pelvic girdle areas. Symptoms usually begin abruptly and it mainly affects women over 50. Severe cases can suffer loss of vision, stroke and migraines due to involvement of the cranial arteries.

Polymyositis

An autoimmune, inflammatory muscle disease of unknown aetiology causing progressive weakness of skeletal muscle. The muscles of the shoulder girdle, hip and pelvis are most commonly affected, although, less commonly, the distal musculature or swallowing can be affected. The muscles can ache and be tender to touch. The disease sometimes occurs with a skin rash over the upper body and is known as dermatomyositis.

Rheumatoid arthritis

Thought to be an autoimmune disease involving the synovium, often affecting several joints at the same time. The joints are affected symmetrically and eventually there is destruction of articular cartilage, capsule, ligaments and tendons, leading to deformity. Clinical features include stiffness, pain, swelling, heat, loss of movement and function. Other manifestations of the disease include subcutaneous nodules, osteoporosis, vasculitis, muscle weakness, fatigue and anaemia. The disease is more common in young to middle-aged women.

Spondylolisthesis

A spontaneous forward displacement of one vertebral body upon the segment below it (usually L5/S1). Displacement may be severe, causing compression of the cauda equina, requiring urgent surgical intervention. Spondylolisthesis is classified according to its cause:

I Dysplastic – congenital
II Isthmic – fatigue fracture of the pars interarticularis due to overuse
III Degenerative – osteoarthritis
IV Traumatic – acute fracture
V Pathological – weakening of the pars interarticularis by a tumour, osteoporosis, tuberculosis or Paget's disease

In rare cases the displacement may be backwards, known as a retrolisthesis.

Spondylolysis

A defect in the pars interarticularis of the lumbar vertebrae (usually L5), often the result of a fatigue fracture. It can be unilateral or bilateral and may or may not progress to spondylolisthesis.

Spondylosis

Degeneration and narrowing of the intervertebral discs leading to the formation of osteophytes at the joint margin and arthritic changes of the facet joints. The lowest three cervical joints are most commonly affected causing neck pain and stiffness, sometimes with radiation to the upper limbs, although the condition may remain symptomless. In some cases osteophytes may encroach sufficiently upon an intervertebral foramen to cause nerve root pressure signs, or, more rarely, the spinal canal to cause dysfunction in all four limbs and possibly the bladder. The vertebral artery can also be involved.

Systemic lupus erythematosus (SLE)

A chronic, inflammatory autoimmune connective tissue disorder involving the skin, joints and internal organs. Clinical features and severity can vary widely depending on the area affected but may include butterfly rash on face, polyarthritis, vasculitis, Raynaud's disease, anaemia, hypertension, neurological disorders, renal disease, pleurisy and alopecia. Of those affected by the disease, around 90% are women.

Systemic sclerosis (scleroderma)

An autoimmune connective tissue disorder that causes an increase in collagen metabolism. Excessive collagen deposits cause damage to microscopic blood vessels in the skin (scleroderma) and other organs (systemic sclerosis), leading to fibrosis and degeneration. Any organ can be affected and its effects can be localized or diffuse, as well as progressive. Middle-aged women are most commonly affected. Clinical features include oedema of hands and feet, contractures and finger deformities, alteration of facial features and dry, shiny, tight skin.

Tennis elbow (lateral epicondylitis)

Tendinopathy of the common origin of the forearm extensors causing pain and tenderness at the lateral aspect of the elbow and down the forearm.

Tenosynovitis

Inflammation of the synovial lining of a tendon sheath caused by mechanical irritation or infection, often associated with overuse and repetitive movements. A similar inflammatory process can affect the paratenon of those tendons without synovial sheaths (peritendinitis).

Tenovaginitis

Inflammatory thickening of the fibrous tendon sheath, sometimes leading to the formation of nodules, usually caused by repeated minor injury. Characterized by restricted movement of the tendon and pain. Common sites to be affected are the flexor sheaths in the fingers or thumb ('trigger' finger) and the sheaths of the extensor pollicis brevis and abductor pollicis longus tendons (de Quervain's syndrome).

Thoracic outlet syndrome

An umbrella term for a group of conditions that result from compression of the neurovascular bundle in the cervicoaxillary canal. Common sites of compression are the costoclavicular space (between the first rib and the clavicle) and the triangle between the anterior scalene, middle scalene and first rib. Causes include muscle shortening and spasm, poor posture, stretching of the lower trunk of the brachial plexus, traumatic structural changes, or, more rarely, congenital anatomical abnormalities such as an enlarged C7 transverse process, cervical rib or clavicular bony abnormality. Clinical features include paraesthesia, pain, subjective weakness, oedema, pallor, discoloration or venous engorgement involving the neck and affected shoulder and upper limb.

Common classifications of fractures

Proximal humeral fractures: Neer's classification

Group I
All proximal humeral fractures where there is minimal displacement or angulation.

Group II
Displaced fractures of the anatomical neck (>1 cm).

Group III
Severely displaced or angled fractures of the surgical neck. These may be impacted or comminuted.

Group IV
Displaced fractures of the greater tuberosity.

Group V
Displaced fractures of the lesser tuberosity.

Group VI
Fracture-dislocations.

Radial head fractures: Hotchkiss modification of Mason's classification

Type 1
Small vertical split with minimal displacement (<2 mm). Stability and rotation largely uncompromised.

Type 2
Displaced single fragment fracture (>2 mm), usually distally. Any fracture that restricts rotation. Any comminuted fracture that can be internally fixated.

Type 3
Highly comminuted fractures that cannot be internally fixated.

Fractures of the radius and ulna

Monteggia fracture-dislocation

Fracture of the ulna associated with dislocation of the radial head.

Galeazzi fracture-dislocation

Fracture of the distal third of the radius associated with dislocation of the inferior radioulnar joint.

Colles' fracture

Transverse fracture of the distal radius with dorsal (posterior) displacement of the distal fragment.

Smith's fracture

Transverse fracture of the distal radius with volar (anterior) displacement of the distal fragment (often called a 'reversed Colles').

Barton's fracture

The true Barton's fracture is a form of Smith's fracture associated with volar subluxation of the carpus. However, dorsal subluxation of the carpus can also occur, which is sometimes called a 'dorsal Barton's fracture'.

Fractures of the thumb metacarpal

Bennett's fracture

Oblique fracture of the first metacarpal extending into the trapezometacarpal joint associated with dislocation of the carpometacarpal joint.

Rolando's fracture

Intra-articular comminuted fracture of the base of the first metacarpal.

Scaphoid fractures: Herbert classification

A1 Fracture of the tubercle (stable)
A2 Hairline fracture of the waist (stable)

B1 Oblique fracture of distal third (unstable)
B2 Displaced fracture of the waist (unstable)
B3 Proximal pole fracture (unstable)
B4 Fracture associated with carpal dislocation (unstable)
B5 Comminuted fracture (unstable)

Pelvic fractures: Tile classification

Type A (stable)

- A1: fractures of the pelvis not involving the pelvic ring
- A2: stable, minimally displaced fractures of the pelvic ring

Type B (rotationally unstable but vertically stable)

- B1: anteroposterior compression fractures (open book fractures)
- B2: lateral compression fractures, ipsilateral
- B3: lateral compression fractures, contralateral

Type C (rotationally and vertically unstable)

- C1: unilateral
- C2: bilateral
- C3: associated with acetabular fracture

Intracapsular fractures of the neck of femur: Garden classification

Type I
Incomplete fracture of the neck of femur with angulation of the trabecular lines.

Type II
Complete fracture without displacement of the neck of femur. The trabecular lines are interrupted but not angulated.

Type III
Complete fracture with partial displacement of the neck of femur.

Type IV

Complete fracture with total displacement of the neck of femur.

Tibial plateau fractures: Schatzker classification

Type I

Split or wedge fracture of the lateral tibial condyle.

Type II

Split or wedge fracture of the lateral tibial condyle combined with depression of the adjacent remaining load-bearing portion of the lateral plateau.

Type III

Pure depression fracture of the lateral tibial plateau without an associated split or wedge fracture.

Type IV

Fracture of the medial tibial plateau. May be a split or a split depression fracture.

Type V

Split fracture of both the medial and lateral tibial condyles.

Type VI

Combined condylar and subcondylar fractures that separate the tibial shaft from the tibial condyles.

Ankle fractures: Weber's classification

Fibular fractures are classified into three types:

Type A

Fracture below the tibiofibular syndesmosis.

Type B

Fracture at the level of the tibial plafond, which often spirals upwards. The syndesmosis is usually involved; however, it remains intact.

Type C

Fracture above the tibiofibular syndesmosis. The syndesmosis is ruptured.

Classification of ligament and muscle sprains

Ligament sprains

Grade I/mild sprain

Few ligament fibres torn, stability maintained.

Grade II/moderate sprain

Partial rupture, increased laxity but no gross instability.

Grade III/severe sprain

Complete rupture, gross instability.

Muscle strains

Grade I/mild strain

Few muscle fibres torn, minimum loss of strength and pain on muscle contraction.

Grade II/moderate strain

Approximately half of muscle fibres torn, significant muscle weakness and loss of function. Moderate to severe pain on isometric contraction.

Grade III/severe strain

Complete tear of the muscle, significant muscle weakness and severe loss of function. Minimum to no pain on isometric contraction.

Common musculoskeletal tests

A concise description of each test is given below. For a fuller description of how each test is performed, please refer to a musculoskeletal assessment textbook (e.g. Gross et al 2002, Magee 2002, Petty & Moore 2002).

Cervical spine

Foramen compression (Spurling's) test

Tests: nerve root compression.

Procedure: patient in sitting. Side flex neck to unaffected side. Carefully apply pressure to top of patient's head. Test is repeated on affected side.

Positive sign: onset or increase in pain radiating into shoulder or arm on side to which head is flexed.

Distraction test

Tests: nerve root compression.

Procedure: patient in sitting. Place one hand under chin and other hand under occiput. Gently lift patient's head.

Positive sign: relief or decrease in pain.

Shoulder

Anterior apprehension (Crank) test

Tests: anterior shoulder stability.

Procedure: patient supine. Gently abduct shoulder to 90°. Gently add lateral rotation.

Positive sign: apprehension.

Anterior drawer test

Tests: anterior shoulder stability.

Procedure: patient supine. Place shoulder in 80–120° abduction, 0–20° forward flexion and 0–30° lateral rotation. Stabilize scapula. Draw humerus anteriorly.

Positive sign: click and/or apprehension.

Clunk test

Tests: tear of glenoid labrum.

Procedure: patient supine. Abduct shoulder over patient's head. Apply anterior force to posterior aspect of humeral head while rotating humerus laterally.

Positive sign: a clunk or grinding sound and/or apprehension if anterior instability present.

Hawkins–Kennedy impingement test

Tests: impingement of supraspinatus tendon.

Procedure: patient sitting or standing. Forward flex shoulder to 90° and flex elbow to 90°. Apply passive medial rotation.

Positive sign: reproduction of symptoms.

Jerk test

Tests: posterior shoulder stability.

Procedure: patient sitting. Place shoulder in 90° forward flexion and medial rotation. Apply longitudinal cephalad force to humerus and move arm into horizontal adduction.

Positive sign: sudden jerk or clunk.

Neer impingement test

Tests: impingement of supraspinatus tendon and/or biceps tendon.

Procedure: patient sitting or standing. Passively elevate arm through forward flexion and medial rotation.

Positive sign: reproduction of symptoms.

Posterior drawer test

Tests: posterior shoulder stability.

Procedure: patient supine. Place shoulder in 100–120° abduction and 20–30° forward flexion with elbow flexed to 120°. Stabilize scapula. Medially rotate and forward flex shoulder between 60 and 80° while pushing head of humerus posteriorly.

Positive sign: significant posterior displacement and/or patient apprehension.

Speed's test

Tests: biceps tendon pathology.

Procedure: patient sitting or standing. Forward flex shoulder, supinate forearm and extend elbow. Resist patient's attempt to flex shoulder.

Positive sign: increased pain in bicipital groove.

Sulcus sign

Tests: inferior shoulder stability.

Procedure: patient standing or sitting, arm by side. Grip arm below elbow and pull distally.

Positive sign: reproduction of symptoms and/or appearance of sulcus under acromion.

Supraspinatus (empty can) test

Tests: supraspinatus tendon pathology; suprascapular nerve neuropathy.

Procedure: patient sitting or standing. Abduct shoulder to 90°. Horizontally flex to 30° and medially rotate so thumbs point downwards. Resist patient's attempt to abduct.

Positive sign: reproduction of symptoms or weakness.

Elbow

Elbow flexion test

Tests: cubital tunnel (ulnar nerve) syndrome.

Procedure: patient standing or sitting. Fully flex elbows with wrist extended. Hold for 5 minutes.

Positive sign: tingling or paraesthesia in ulnar nerve distribution.

Lateral epicondylitis (tennis elbow) test: method 1

Tests: lateral epicondylitis.

Procedure: passively extend elbow, pronate forearm and flex wrist and fingers while palpating lateral epicondyle.

Positive sign: reproduction of symptoms.

Lateral epicondylitis (tennis elbow) test: method 2

Tests: lateral epicondylitis.

Procedure: resist extension of middle finger distal to PIP (proximal interphalangeal) joint.

Positive sign: reproduction of symptoms.

Medial epicondylitis (golfer's elbow) test

Tests: medial epicondylitis.

Procedure: passively extend elbow, supinate forearm and extend wrist and fingers while palpating medial epicondyle.
Positive sign: reproduction of symptoms.

Pinch grip test

Tests: anterior interosseous (median) nerve entrapment.
Procedure: patient pinches tips of index finger and thumb together.
Positive sign: inability to pinch tip to tip.

Tinel's sign (at elbow)

Tests: point of regeneration of sensory fibres of ulnar nerve.
Procedure: tap ulnar nerve in groove between olecranon and medial epicondyle.
Positive sign: tingling sensation in ulnar distribution of forearm and hand. Furthest point at which abnormal sensation felt indicates point to which the nerve has regenerated.

Varus stress test

Tests: stability of lateral collateral ligament.
Procedure: patient in sitting. Stabilize upper arm with elbow in 20–30° flexion and humerus in full medial rotation. Apply adduction/varus force to forearm.
Positive sign: excessive laxity or reproduction of symptoms.

Valgus stress test

Tests: stability of medial collateral ligament.
Procedure: patient in sitting. Stabilize upper arm with elbow in 20–30° flexion and humerus in full lateral rotation. Apply abduction/valgus force to forearm.
Positive sign: increased laxity or reproduction of symptoms.

Wrist and hand

Finkelstein test

Tests: tenosynovitis of abductor pollicis longus and extensor pollicis brevis tendons (de Quervain's tenosynovitis).

Procedure: patient makes a fist with thumb inside. Passively move wrist into ulnar deviation.

Positive sign: reproduction of symptoms.

Froment's sign

Tests: ulnar nerve paralysis.

Procedure: grip piece of paper between index finger and thumb. Pull paper away.

Positive sign: flexion of IP (interphalangeal) thumb joint as paper pulled away.

Ligamentous instability test for the fingers

Tests: stability of collateral ligaments.

Procedure: apply valgus and varus force to PIP (proximal interphalangeal) or DIP (distal interphalangeal) joint.

Positive sign: increased laxity.

Linburg's sign

Tests: tendon pathology at interconnection between flexor pollicis longus and flexor indices.

Procedure: thumb flexion onto hypothenar eminence and index finger extension.

Positive sign: limited extension and reproduction of symptoms.

Lunotriquetral ballottement (Reagan's) test

Tests: stability of lunotriquetral ligament.

Procedure: stabilize triquetrum and apply posterior and anterior glide to lunate.

Positive sign: reproduction of symptoms, crepitus or laxity.

Phalen's (wrist flexion) test

Tests: median nerve pathology; carpal tunnel syndrome.

Procedure: place dorsal aspect of hands together with wrists flexed. Hold for 1 minute.

Positive sign: tingling in distribution of median nerve.

Reverse Phalen's test

Tests: median nerve pathology.

Procedure: place palms of hands together with wrists extended. Hold for 1 minute.
Positive sign: tingling in distribution of median nerve.

Sweater finger sign

Tests: rupture of flexor digitorum profundus tendon.
Procedure: patient makes a fist.
Positive sign: loss of DIP joint flexion of one of the fingers.

Tinel's sign (at the wrist)

Tests: median nerve pathology; carpal tunnel syndrome.
Procedure: tap over carpal tunnel.
Positive sign: tingling or paraesthesia in median distribution in hand. Furthest point at which abnormal sensation felt indicates point to which the nerve has regenerated.

Watson (scaphoid shift) test

Tests: stability of scaphoid.
Procedure: hold wrist in full ulnar deviation and slight extension. With other hand apply pressure to scaphoid tubercle (palmar aspect) and move wrist into radial deviation and slight flexion.
Positive sign: pain and/or subluxation of scaphoid.

Pelvis

Anterior gapping test

Tests: sprain of anterior sacroiliac joint or ligaments.
Procedure: patient supine. Push right and left ASIS (anterior superior iliac spine) apart.
Positive sign: reproduction of symptoms.

Gillet's test

Tests: sacroiliac joint dysfunction.
Procedure: patient standing. Palpate PSIS (posterior superior iliac spine) and sacrum at same level. Patient flexes hip and knee on side being palpated while standing on opposite leg. Repeat test on other side and compare.

Positive sign: if the PSIS on the side tested does not move downwards in relation to the sacrum it indicates hypomobility on that side.

Hibb's test

Tests: movement of sacroiliac joint, stresses posterior sacroiliac ligaments.

Procedure: patient prone. Stabilize pelvis and flex knee to 90°. Medially rotate hip while palpating sacroiliac joint on that side. Repeat test on other side.

Positive sign: difference in amount of opening and quality of movement at each sacroiliac joint.

Piedallu's sign (sitting flexion)

Tests: movement of sacrum on ilia.

Procedure: patient sitting. Left and right PSIS are palpated while patient forward flexes.

Positive sign: one side moves higher than the other, indicating hypomobility on that side.

Posterior gapping test

Tests: sprain of posterior sacroiliac joint or ligaments.

Procedure: patient supine or side lying. Push right and left ASIS towards each other.

Positive sign: reproduction of symptoms.

Supine to sit (long sitting) test

Tests: pelvic torsion or rotation.

Procedure: patient supine. Note level of inferior borders of medial malleoli. Patient sits up and relative position of malleoli noted.

Positive sign: one leg moves up more than the other.

Standing flexion

Tests: movement of ilia on sacrum.

Procedure: patient standing. Left and right PSIS are palpated while patient forward flexes.

Positive sign: one side moves higher than the other, indicating hypomobility on that side.

Hip

Faber's test (Patrick's test)

Tests: hip joint or sacroiliac joint dysfunction; spasm of iliopsoas muscle.

Procedure: patient supine. Place foot of test leg on opposite knee. Gently lower knee of test leg.

Positive sign: knee remains above the opposite leg; pain or spasm.

Ober's sign

Tests: tensor fascia lata and iliotibial band contractures.

Procedure: patient in side lying with hip and knee of lower leg flexed. Stabilize pelvis. Passively abduct and extend upper leg with knee extended or flexed to 90°, then allow it to drop towards plinth.

Positive sign: upper leg remains abducted and does not lower to plinth.

Rectus femoris contracture test

Tests: rectus femoris contracture.

Procedure: patient supine with test knee flexed to 90° over edge of plinth. Patient hugs other knee to chest.

Positive sign: knee over edge of plinth extends.

Thomas test

Tests: hip flexion contracture.

Procedure: patient supine. Patient hugs one knee to chest.

Positive sign: opposite leg lifts off plinth.

Trendelenburg's sign

Tests: stability of the hip, strength of hip abductors (gluteus medius).

Procedure: patient stands on one leg.

Positive sign: pelvis on opposite side drops.

Knee

Abduction (valgus) stress test

Tests: full knee extension: anterior cruciate ligament, medial quadriceps expansion, semimembranosus muscle, medial collateral ligaments, posterior oblique ligament, posterior cruciate ligament, posteromedial capsule.

20–30° flexion: medial collateral ligament, posterior oblique ligament, posterior cruciate ligament, posteromedial capsule.

Procedure: patient supine. Stabilize ankle and apply medial pressure (valgus stress) to knee joint at 0° and then at 20–30° extension.

Positive sign: excessive movement compared to opposite knee.

Adduction (varus) stress test

Tests: full knee extension: cruciate ligaments, lateral gastrocnemius muscle, lateral collateral ligament, arcuate–popliteus complex, posterolateral capsule, iliotibial band, biceps femoris tendon.

20–30° flexion: lateral collateral ligament, arcuate–popliteus complex, posterolateral capsule, iliotibial band, biceps femoris tendon.

Procedure: patient supine. Stabilize ankle. Apply lateral pressure (varus stress) to knee joint at 0° and then at 20–30° extension.

Positive sign: excessive movement compared to opposite knee.

Anterior drawer test

Tests: anterior cruciate ligament, posterior oblique ligament, arcuate–popliteus complex, posteromedial and posterolateral capsules, medial collateral ligament, iliotibial band.

Procedure: patient supine with hips flexed to 45° and knee flexed to 90°. Stabilize foot. Apply posteroanterior force to tibia.

Positive sign: tibia moves more than 6 mm on the femur.

Apley's test

Tests: distraction for ligamentous injury; compression for meniscus injury.

Procedure: patient prone with knee flexed to 90°. Medially and laterally rotate tibia – first with distraction and then compression.

Positive sign: pain.

Brush test

Tests: mild effusion.

Procedure: stroke medial side of patella from just below joint line up to suprapatellar pouch two or three times. Use opposite hand to stroke down lateral side of patella.

Positive sign: fluid travels to medial side and appears as bulge below distal border of patella.

External rotation recurvatum test

Tests: posterolateral rotary stability in knee extension.

Procedure: patient supine. Hold heel and place knee in 30° flexion. Slowly extend knee while palpating posterolateral aspect of knee.

Positive sign: excessive hyperextension and lateral rotation palpated.

Fairbank's apprehension test

Tests: patellar subluxation or dislocation.

Procedure: patient supine with knee in 30° flexion and quads relaxed. Passively glide patella laterally.

Positive sign: patient apprehension or excessive movement.

Hughston plica test

Tests: inflammation of suprapatellar plica.

Procedure: patient supine. Flex and medially rotate knee while applying medial glide to patella and palpating medial femoral condyle. Passively extend and flex knee.

Positive sign: popping of plica band over femoral condyle, tenderness.

Lachman's test

Tests: anterior cruciate ligament, posterior oblique ligament, arcuate–popliteus complex.

Procedure: patient supine with knee flexed 0–30°. Stabilize femur. Apply posteroanterior force to tibia.

Positive sign: soft end feel or excessive movement.

McConnell test for chondromalacia patellae

Tests: chondromalacia patellae.

Procedure: patient in high sitting with femur laterally rotated. Isometric quad contractions are performed at 0°, 30°, 60°, 90° and 120° of knee flexion for 10 seconds. If pain is produced with any of these movements, repeat test with patella pushed medially.

Positive sign: decrease in symptoms with medial glide.

McMurray test

Tests: medial meniscus and lateral meniscus injury.

Procedure: patient supine with test knee completely flexed. To test the medial meniscus, laterally rotate knee and passively extend to 90° while palpating joint line. To test the lateral meniscus, repeat test with the knee in medial rotation.

Positive sign: a snap or click.

Posterior drawer test

Tests: posterior cruciate ligament, arcuate–popliteus complex, posterior oblique ligament, anterior cruciate ligament.

Procedure: patient supine with hips flexed to 45° and knee flexed to 90°. Stabilize foot. Apply anteroposterior force to tibia.

Positive sign: excessive movement.

Posterior sag sign

Tests: posterior cruciate ligament, arcuate–popliteus complex, posterior oblique ligament, anterior cruciate ligament.

Procedure: patient supine with hips flexed to 45° and knee flexed to 90° with feet on plinth.

Positive sign: tibia drops posteriorly.

Slocum test for anterolateral rotary instability

Tests: anterior and posterior cruciate ligaments, posterolateral capsule, arcuate–popliteus complex, lateral collateral ligaments, iliotibial band.

Procedure: patient supine with hips flexed to 45° and knee flexed to 90°. Place foot in 30° medial rotation and stabilize. Apply posteroanterior force to tibia.

Positive sign: excessive movement on lateral side when compared with other knee.

Slocum test for anteromedial rotary instability

Tests: medial collateral ligament, posterior oblique ligament, posteromedial capsule, anterior cruciate ligament.

Procedure: patient supine with hips flexed to 45° and knee flexed to 90°. Place foot in 15° lateral rotation and stabilize. Apply posteroanterior force to tibia.

Positive sign: excessive movement on medial side when compared with other knee.

Ankle and foot

Anterior drawer sign

Tests: medial and lateral ligament integrity.

Procedure: patient prone with knee flexed. Apply posteroanterior force to talus with ankle in dorsiflexion and then plantarflexion.

Positive sign: excessive anterior movement (both ligaments affected) or movement on one side only (ligament on that side affected).

Talar tilt

Tests: adduction: mainly integrity of calcaneofibular ligament but also anterior talofibular ligament. Abduction: integrity of deltoid ligament.

Procedure: patient prone, supine or side lying with knee flexed. Tilt talus into abduction and adduction with patient's foot in neutral.

Positive sign: excessive movement.

Thompson's test

Tests: Achilles tendon rupture.

Procedure: patient prone with feet over edge of plinth. Squeeze calf muscles.

Positive sign: absence of plantarflexion.

Common vascular tests

Adson's manoeuvre

Tests: thoracic outlet syndrome.

Procedure: patient sitting. Patient turns head towards test arm and extends head. Laterally rotate and extend shoulder and arm while palpating radial pulse. Patient takes a deep breath and holds it.

Positive sign: disappearance of radial pulse.

Allen manoeuvre

Tests: thoracic outlet syndrome.

Procedure: patient sitting with shoulder abducted to 90°, horizontally extended and laterally rotated and elbow flexed. Palpate radial pulse while patient turns head away from test side.

Positive sign: disappearance of radial pulse.

Homan's test

Tests: deep vein thrombophlebitis.

Procedure: patient supine. Passive dorsiflexion of ankle with knee extended.

Positive sign: pain in the calf.

Provocation elevation test

Tests: thoracic outlet syndrome.

Procedure: patient standing with arms above head. Opens and closes hands 15 times.

Positive sign: fatigue, cramp, tingling.

Vertebral artery test

Tests: vertebrobasilar insufficiency.

Procedure: patient sitting or supine. Patient performs each of the movements listed below actively. Maintain position with gentle overpressure for a minimum of 10 seconds with a 10-second break before the next movement is performed. The movements are increasingly provocative and the test should be stopped if symptoms occur.

Movements:

1 Sustained cervical extension
2 Sustained left and right cervical rotation
3 Sustained left and right cervical rotation with extension
4 Position that provokes symptoms
5 Quick head movement into provocative position
6 Quick repeated head movement into provocative position
7 Sustained trunk movements to left and right while head remains still
8 Repeated trunk movements to left and right while head remains still.

Positive sign: nystagmus, visual disturbances, dizziness, light-headedness.

Signs and symptoms that may indicate possible vertebral–basilar artery problems (from Magee 2002, with permission of Elsevier)

Signs and symptoms

- Malaise and nausea
- Vomiting
- Dizziness/vertigo
- Unsteadiness in walking, incoordination
- Visual disturbances
- Severe headaches
- Weakness in extremities
- Sensory changes in face or body
- Dysarthria
- Unconsciousness, disorientation, light-headedness
- Dysphagia
- Hearing difficulties
- Facial paralysis

Neurodynamic tests (from Petty & Moore 2002, with permission)

Upper limb tension tests

When conducting the upper limb tension tests (ULTT) the sequence of the test movements is relatively unimportant and may be adapted to suit the patient's condition. However, if the tests are to be of value as an assessment tool, the order used for a particular patient must be the same each time the patient is tested.

ULTT 1

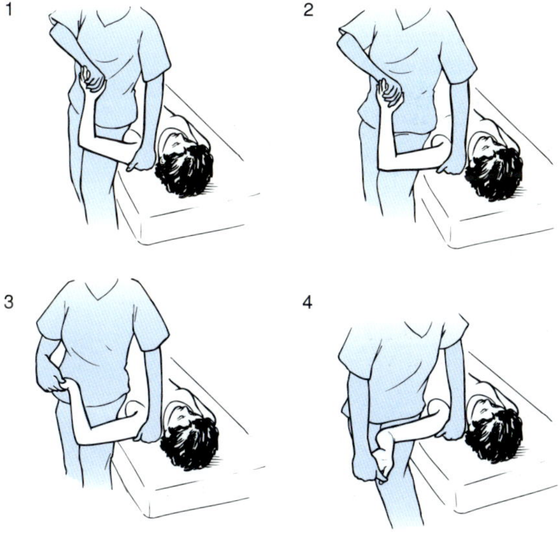

Figure 1.34 (1–6) Upper limb tension test 1.

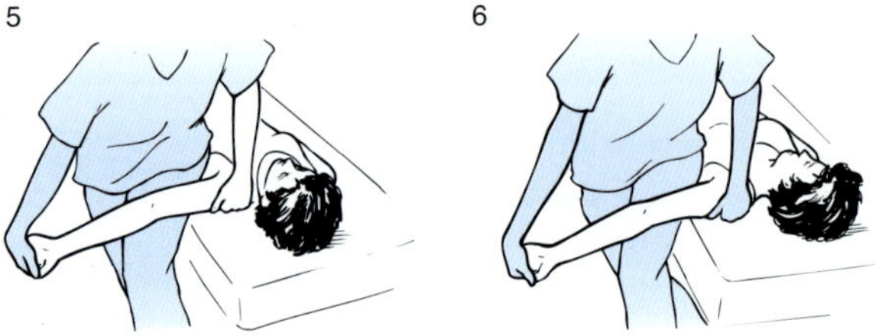

Figure 1.34 (*Continued*).

ULTT 1 consists of:

- Fixing shoulder to prevent shoulder elevation during abduction (Fig. 1.34[1])
- Shoulder joint abduction (Fig. 1.34[2])
- Wrist and finger extension (Fig. 1.34[3])
- Forearm supination (Fig. 1.34[3])
- Shoulder lateral rotation (Fig. 1.34[4])
- Elbow extension (Fig. 1.34[5])

Sensitizing test: cervical lateral flexion away from the symptomatic side (Fig. 1.34[6]).

Desensitizing test: cervical lateral flexion towards the symptomatic side.

ULTT 2a

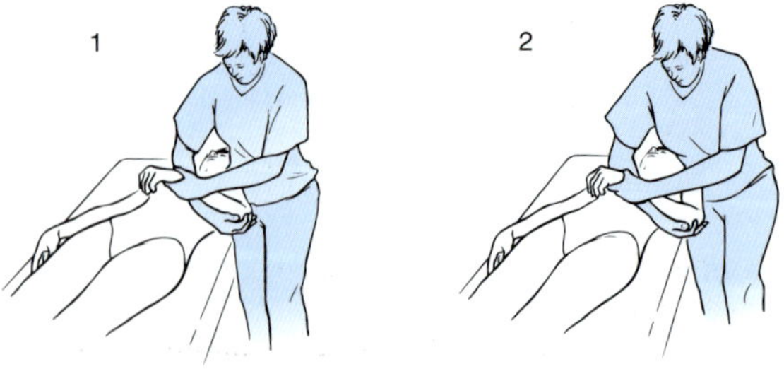

Figure 1.35 (1–6) Upper limb tension test 2a. Median nerve bias.

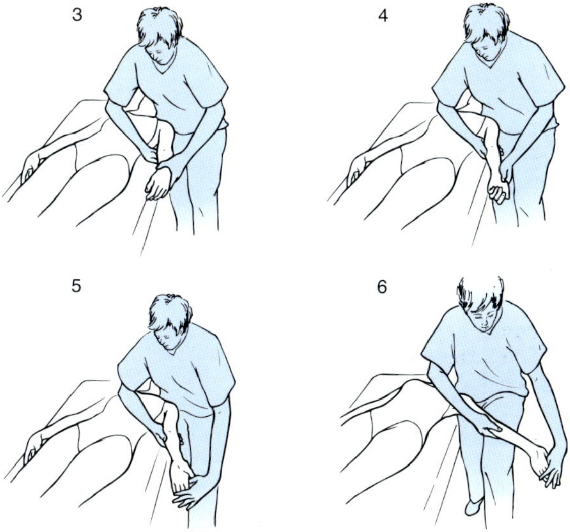

Figure 1.35 (*Continued*).

ULTT 2a consists of:

- Shoulder girdle depression with approximately 10° shoulder joint abduction (Figs 1.35[1],[2])
- Elbow extension (Fig. 1.35[3])
- Lateral rotation of whole arm (Fig. 1.35[4])
- Wrist, finger and thumb extension (Fig. 1.35[5])
- Abduction of shoulder (Fig. 1.35[6])

Sensitizing test: cervical lateral flexion away from the symptomatic side.

Desensitizing tests: cervical lateral flexion towards the symptomatic side or release of the shoulder girdle depression.

ULTT 2b

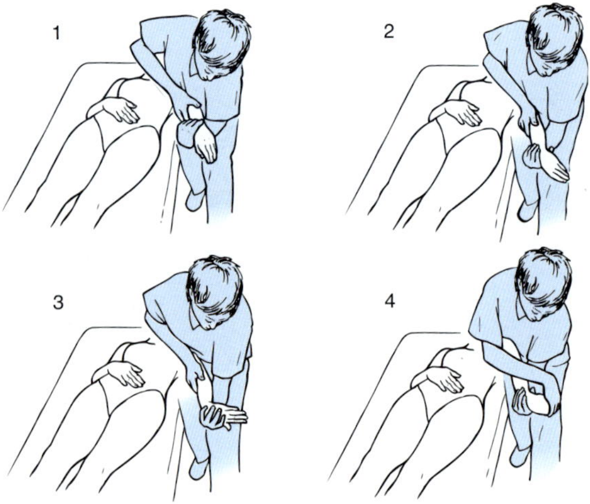

Figure 1.36 (1–4) Upper limb tension test 2b. Radial nerve bias.

ULTT 2b consists of:

- Shoulder girdle depression with about 10° shoulder joint abduction (Fig. 1.36[1])
- Elbow extension (Fig. 1.36[2])
- Medial rotation of whole arm (Fig. 1.36[3])
- Wrist flexion (Fig. 1.36[4])

To further load the radial nerve add thumb flexion and ulnar deviation.

Sensitizing test: cervical lateral flexion away from the symptomatic side.

Desensitizing tests: cervical lateral flexion towards the symptomatic side or release of the shoulder girdle depression.

ULTT 3

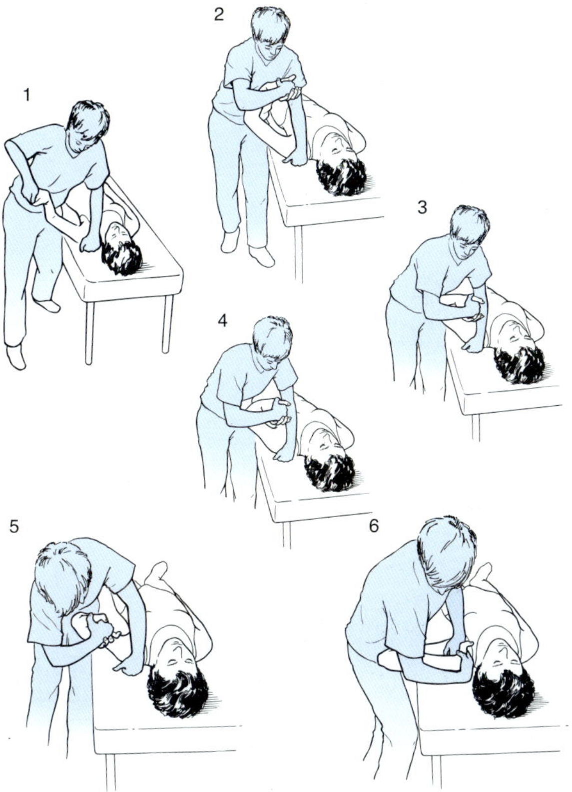

Figure 1.37 (1–6) Upper limb tension test 3. Ulnar nerve bias.

ULTT 3 consists of:

- Wrist and finger extension (Fig. 1.37[1])
- Forearm pronation (Fig. 1.37[2])
- Elbow flexion (Fig. 1.37[3])
- Shoulder lateral rotation (Fig. 1.37[4])
- Shoulder girdle depression (Fig. 1.37[5])
- Shoulder abduction (Fig. 1.37[6])

Slump test

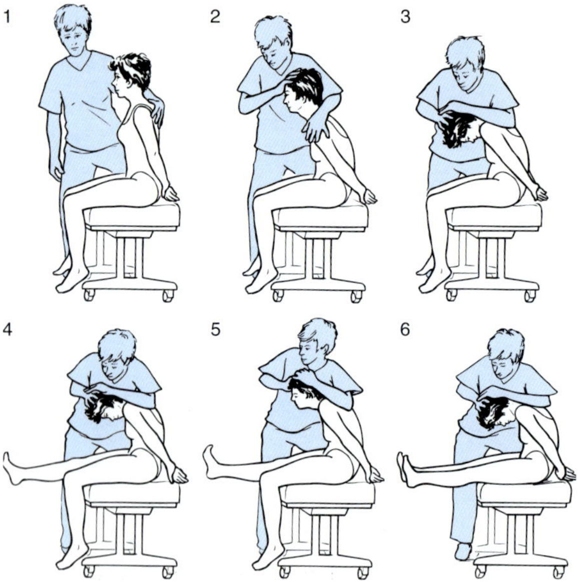

Figure 1.38 (1–6) Slump test.

Starting position: patient sits upright with knee crease at the edge of plinth and hands behind back (Fig. 1.38[1]).

The slump test consists of:

- Spinal slump (Fig. 1.38[2])
- Neck flexion (Fig. 1.38[3])
- Knee extension (Fig. 1.38[4])
- Release neck flexion (Fig. 1.38[5])

The steps can be performed in any order.

Additional movements: add dorsiflexion or plantarflexion with knee extension; bilateral knee extension (Fig. 1.38[6]).

Straight leg raise

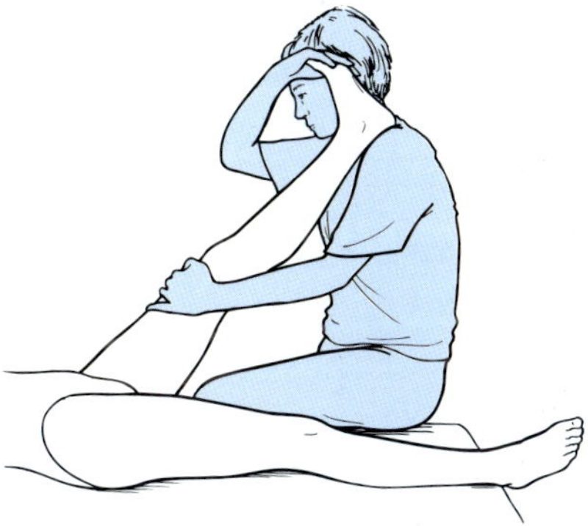

Figure 1.39 Straight leg raise.

The test consists of passive hip flexion with the knee extended.

Sensitizing tests: add ankle dorsiflexion and eversion, plantarflexion and inversion, hip adduction, hip medial rotation, neck flexion and spinal lateral flexion.

Passive neck flexion

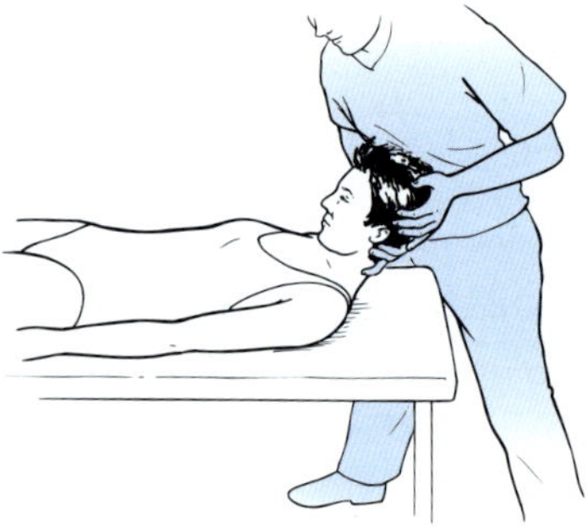

Figure 1.40 Passive neck flexion.

The test consists of passive neck flexion.

Sensitizing tests: straight leg raise, upper limb tension tests.

Slump knee bend

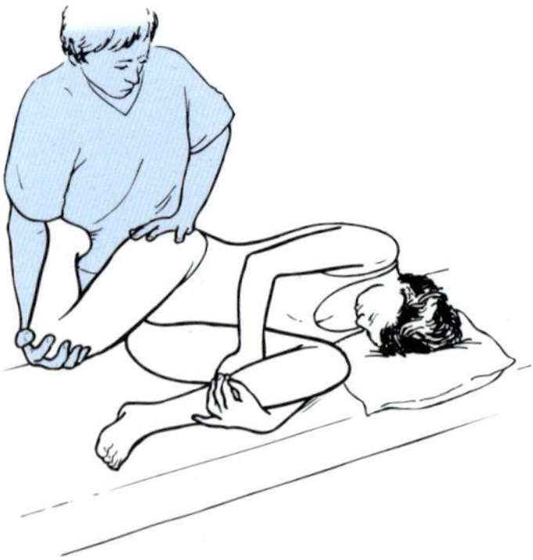

Figure 1.41 Slump knee bend.

Starting position: patient in side lying. Holds bottom knee to chest and flexes neck.

The slump knee bend consists of:

1 Flex uppermost knee
2 Hip extension

Desensitizing test: cervical extension.

Precautions with physical neural examination and management (from Butler 2000 *The Sensitive Nervous System*, Noigroup Press, with permission of Noigroup Publications)

- Patients with suspected 'red flags' need to be identified and managed accordingly
- Take care with elongation and pinching manoeuvres with acute nerve root disorders
- Watch that repeated movements do not aggravate a central sensitivity state
- Be careful in acute states, when clinical pictures such as disc trauma or compartment syndrome suggests that nerve irritation/compression could occur
- Take care with recent apparent peripheral severe nerve injury that may, initially, be clinically silent. Wait for a few days to see what the clinical expression will be
- There are some states where peripheral nerves appear tethered and will not move with various physical therapies. Repeated attempts will just worsen the problem. A surgical opinion is necessary
- Take care with disorders such as diabetes, rheumatoid arthritis and Guillain–Barré. However, programmes including graded mobilization and fitness may be useful for symptomatic relief and to minimize complications
- Where there are hard upper motor neurone signs, as could occur after trauma or with tethered cord syndrome, seek specialist medical opinion

Diagnostic triage for back pain (including red flags) (from Clinical Standards Advisory Group 1994, with permission)

The main diagnostic indicators for simple backache, nerve root pain and possible serious spinal pathology ('red flags') are outlined below:

Simple backache

- Onset generally age 20–55 years
- Lumbosacral region, buttocks and thighs
- Pain mechanical in nature
  - varies with physical activity
  - varies with time
- Patient well
- Prognosis good (90% recover from acute attack in 6 weeks)

Nerve root pain

- Unilateral leg pain > back pain
- Pain generally radiates to foot or toes
- Numbness and paraesthesia in the same distribution
- Nerve irritation signs
  - reduced straight leg raising which reproduces leg pain
- Motor, sensory or reflex change
  - limited to one nerve root
- Prognosis reasonable
  - (50% recover from acute attack within 6 weeks)

Possible serious spinal pathology

Red flags

- Age of onset <20 or >55 years
- Violent trauma: e.g. fall from a height, road traffic accident
- Constant, progressive, non-mechanical pain

- Thoracic pain
- PMH – carcinoma
- Systemic steroids
- Drug abuse, HIV
- Systemically unwell
- Weight loss
- Persisting severe restriction of lumbar flexion
- Widespread neurology
- Structural deformity

If there are suspicious clinical features, or if pain has not settled in 6 weeks, an ESR and plain X-ray should be considered.

Cauda equina syndrome/widespread neurological disorder

- Difficulty with micturition
- Loss of anal sphincter tone or faecal incontinence
- Saddle anaesthesia about the anus, perineum or genitals
- Widespread (>one nerve root) or progressive motor weakness in the legs or gait disturbance

Inflammatory disorders (ankylosing spondylitis and related disorders)

- Gradual onset
- Marked morning stiffness
- Persisting limitation of spinal movements in all directions
- Peripheral joint involvement
- Iritis, skin rashes (psoriasis), colitis, urethral discharge
- Family history

Yellow flags

Risk factors for chronicity (Clinical Standards Advisory Group 1994, with permission)

- Previous history of low back pain
- Total work loss (due to low back pain) in past 12 months
- Radiating leg pain

- Reduced straight leg raising
- Signs of nerve root involvement
- Reduced muscle strength and endurance
- Poor physical fitness
- Self-rated health poor
- Heavy smoking
- Psychological distress and depressive symptoms
- Disproportionate illness behaviour
- Low job satisfaction
- Personal problems – alcohol, marital, financial
- Adversarial medico-legal proceedings

Low educational attainment and heavy physical occupation slightly increase the risk of low back pain and chronicity but markedly increase the difficulty of rehabilitation and retraining.

Main categories for psychosocial yellow flags (Waddell 1998)

Attitudes and beliefs about back pain
Behaviours
Compensation issues
Diagnostic and treatment issues
Emotions
Family
Work

Musculoskeletal assessment (based on Petty & Moore 2002, with permission)

Patients present with a variety of conditions and assessments need to be adapted to suit their needs. This chapter provides a basic framework for the subjective and physical musculoskeletal assessment of a patient.

Subjective examination

Body chart

Type and area of current symptoms
Depth, quality, intensity of symptoms
Intermittent or constant
Abnormal sensation (e.g. pins and needles, numbness)
Relationship of symptoms
Check other relevant regions

Behaviour of symptoms

Aggravating factors
Easing factors
Severity
Irritability
Daily activities/functional limitations
24-hour behaviour
Stage of the condition

Special questions

General health
THREAD (Thyroid disorders, Heart problems, Rheumatoid arthritis, Epilepsy, Asthma or other respiratory problems, Diabetes)
Drugs
Steroids
Anticoagulants
Recent unexplained weight loss
Spinal cord or cauda equina symptoms
Dizziness or other symptoms of vertebrobasilar insufficiency
Recent X-rays or investigations

History of present condition

History of each symptomatic area
Relationship of onset of each symptomatic area
Change of each symptom since onset

Past medical history

Relevant medical history
Previous episodes of present complaint
Previous treatment and outcome

Social and family history

Age and gender
Home and work situation
Dependants
Leisure activities
Yellow flags

Physical examination

Observation

Formal and informal observation of posture and function
Muscle bulk and tone
Soft tissues

Active and passive joint movements

Active and passive physiological movements
Joint integrity tests
Joint effusion measurement

Muscle tests

Muscle strength
Muscle control and stability
Muscle length
Isometric muscle testing

Neurological tests

Integrity of the nervous system
- dermatomes
- reflexes
- myotomes

Mobility of the nervous system
- straight leg raise
- slump test

- prone knee bend
- passive neck flexion
- upper limb tension tests

Special tests (e.g. coordination)

Special tests

Vascular tests
Measurement of bony abnormality
Soft tissue tests

Palpation

Skin and superficial soft tissue
Muscle and tendon
Nerve
Ligament
Joint
Bone

Passive accessory movements

References and further reading

Adams J C, Hamblen D L 2001 Outline of orthopaedics, 13th edn. Churchill Livingstone, Edinburgh

Baxter R 1998 Pocket guide to musculoskeletal assessment. W B Saunders, Philadelphia

Brukner P, Khan K 2001 Clinical sports medicine, 2nd edn. McGraw-Hill, Sydney

Butler D S 2000 The sensitive nervous system. Noigroup Publications, Adelaide

Clinical Standards Advisory Group 1994 Back pain: report of a CSAG committee on back pain. HMSO, London

Cyriax J 1982 Textbook of orthopaedic medicine. Vol. 1: Diagnosis of soft tissue lesions, 8th edn. Baillière Tindall, London

Dandy D J, Edwards D J 1998 Essential orthopaedics and trauma, 3rd edn. Churchill Livingstone, Edinburgh

David C, Lloyd J 1998 Rheumatological physiotherapy. Mosby, London

Grieve G P 1991 Mobilisation of the spine: a primary handbook of clinical method, 5th edn. Churchill Livingstone, Edinburgh

Gross J, Fetto J, Rosen E 2002 Musculoskeletal examination, 2nd edn. Blackwell Science, Malden, MA

Kendall F P, McCreary E K, Provance P G 1993 Muscles: testing and function, 4th edn. Williams and Wilkins, Baltimore

Kitchen S 2002 Electrotherapy: evidence-based practice, 11th edn. Churchill Livingstone, Edinburgh

McRae R 1999 Pocketbook of orthopaedics and fractures. Churchill Livingstone, Edinburgh

McRae R, Esser M 2002 Practical fracture treatment, 4th edn. Churchill Livingstone, Edinburgh

Magee D J 2002 Orthopaedic physical assessment, 4th edn. Saunders, Philadelphia

Maitland G D 1991 Peripheral manipulation, 3rd edn. Butterworth-Heinemann, Oxford

Maitland G D 2001 Maitland's vertebral manipulation. Butterworth-Heinemann, Oxford

O'Brian M D 2000 Guarantors of 'Brain' 1999–2000 (prepared by O'Brian M D). Aids to the examination of the peripheral nervous system. W B Saunders, Edinburgh

Ombregt L, Bisschop P 1999 Atlas of orthopaedic examination of the peripheral joints. W B Saunders, Edinburgh

Palastanga N, Field D, Soames R 2002 Anatomy and human movement: structure and function, 4th edn. Butterworth-Heinemann, Oxford

Petty N J, Moore A P 2002 Neuromusculoskeletal examination and assessment: a handbook for therapists, 2nd edn. Churchill Livingstone, Edinburgh

Rothstein J M, Roy S H, Wolf S L 1998 The rehabilitation specialist's handbook, 2nd edn. F A Davis, Philadelphia

Soloman L, Warwick D J, Nayagam S 2001 Apley's system of orthopaedics and fractures, 8th edn. Arnold, London

Stone R J, Stone J A 2002 Atlas of skeletal muscles, 4th edn. McGraw-Hill, Boston

Waddell G 1998 The back pain revolution. Churchill Livingstone, Edinburgh

Williams P L 1995 Gray's anatomy, 38th edn. Churchill Livingstone, Edinburgh

SECTION 2

Neurology

Neuroanatomy illustrations

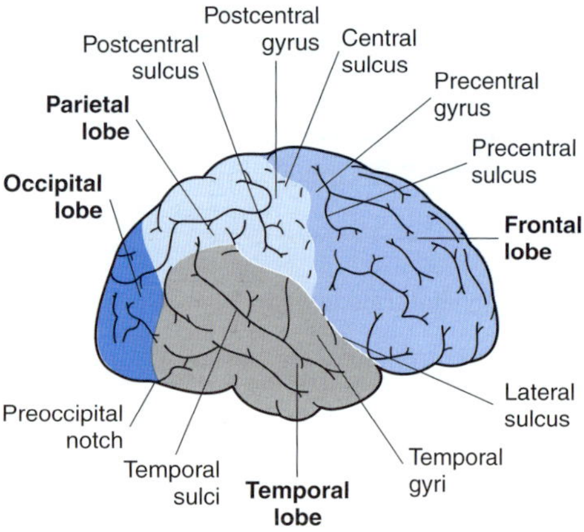

Figure 2.1 Lateral view of right cerebral hemisphere.

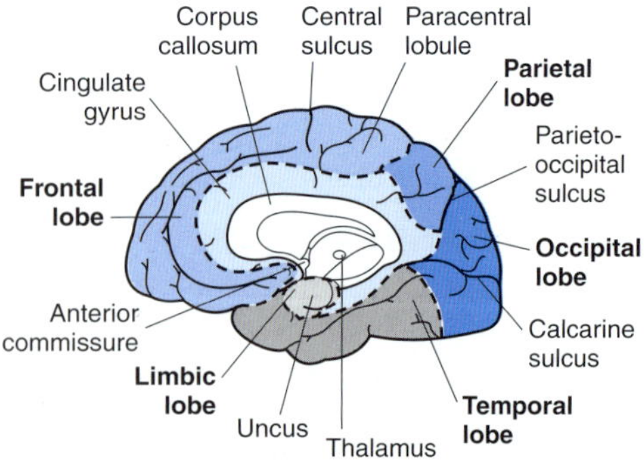

Figure 2.2 Medial view of right cerebral hemisphere.

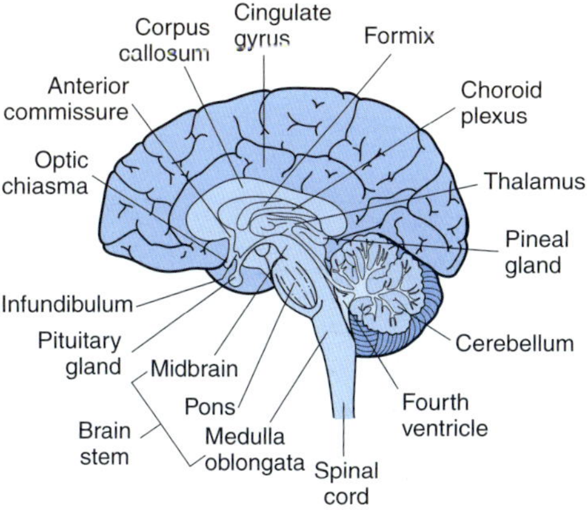

Figure 2.3 Mid-sagittal section of the brain.

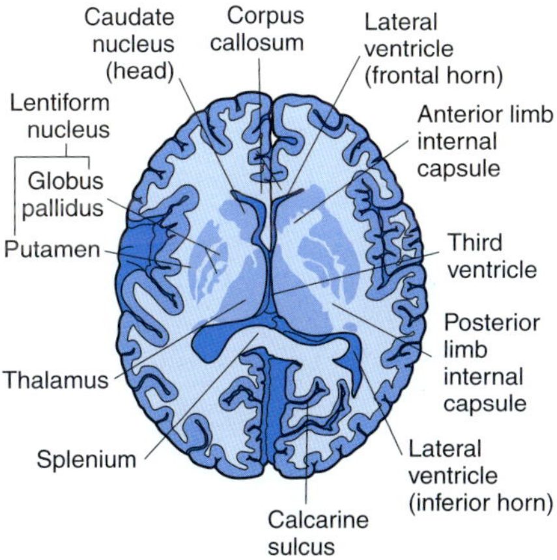

Figure 2.4 Horizontal section through the brain.

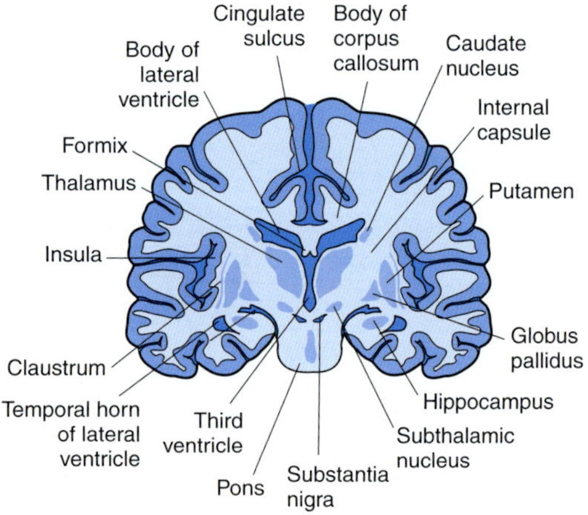

Figure 2.5 Coronal section of the brain.

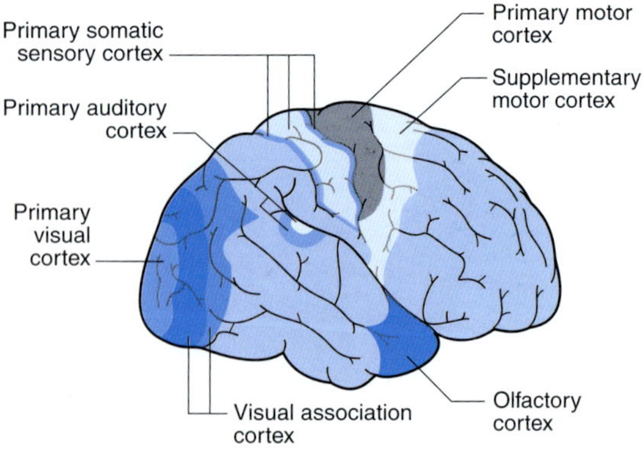

Figure 2.6 Lateral view of sensory and motor cortical areas.

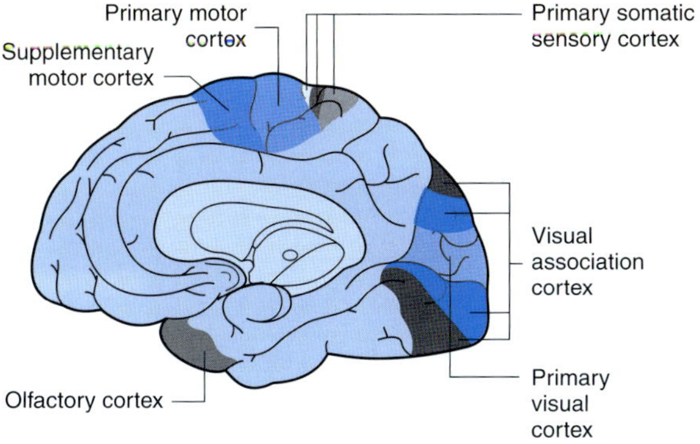

Figure 2.7 Medial view of sensory and motor cortical areas.

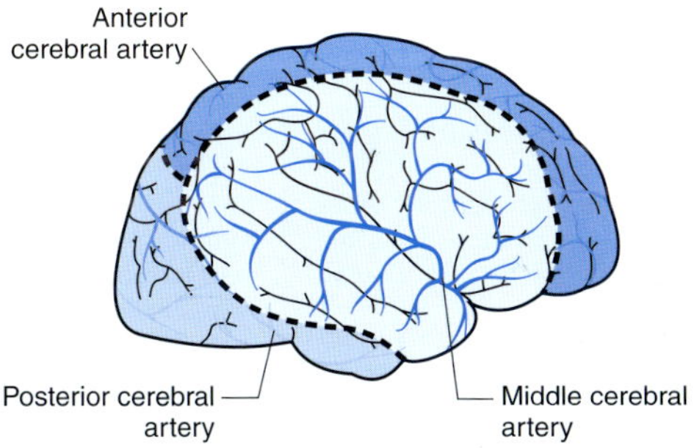

Figure 2.8 Lateral view of right hemisphere showing territories supplied by the cerebral arteries.

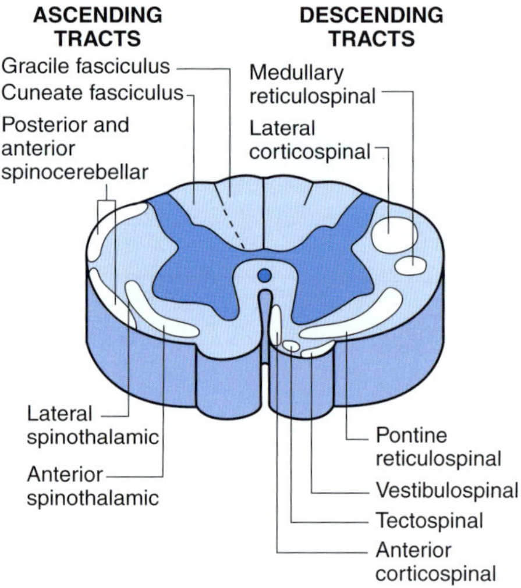

Ascending tracts	Descending tracts
Gracile fasciculus – proprioception and discriminative touch in legs and lower trunk Cuneate fasciculus – proprioception and discriminative touch in arms and upper trunk Posterior and anterior spinocerebellar – reflex and proprioception Lateral spinothalamic – pain and temperature Anterior spinothalamic – light touch	Lateral corticospinal – voluntary movements Medullary retrospinal – locomotion and posture Pontine reticulospinal – locomotion and posture Vestibulospinal – balance and antigravity muscles Tectospinal – orientates head to visual stimulation Anterior corticospinal – voluntary movements

Figure 2.9 Ascending and descending spinal cord tracts.

Signs and symptoms of cerebrovascular lesions

Middle cerebral artery (MCA)

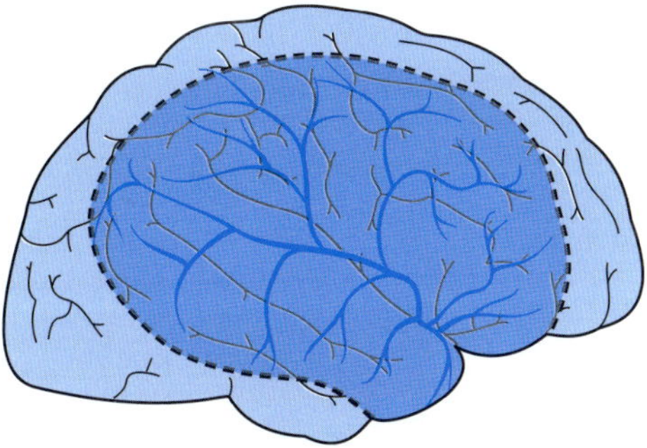

Figure 2.10 Middle cerebral artery.

The middle cerebral artery arises from the internal carotid artery. The proximal part supplies a large portion of the frontal, parietal and temporal lobes. The deep branches supply the basal ganglia (corpus striatum and globus pallidus), internal capsule and thalamus.

Signs and symptoms	Structures involved
Contralateral weakness/paralysis of face, arm, trunk and leg	Motor cortex (precentral gyrus)
Contralateral sensory impairment/loss of face, arm, trunk and leg	Somatosensory cortex (postcentral gyrus)
Broca's dysphasia	Motor speech area of Broca (dominant frontal lobe)
Wernicke's dysphasia	Sensory speech area of Wernicke (dominant parietal/temporal lobe)

Signs and symptoms	Structures involved
Neglect of contralateral side, dressing and constructional apraxia, geographical agnosia, anosognosia	Parietal lobe (non-dominant lobe)
Homonymous hemianopia (often upper homonymous quadrantanopia)	Optic radiation – temporal fibres
Ocular deviation	Frontal lobe
Gait disturbance	Frontal lobe (usually bilateral)
Pure motor hemiplegia	Posterior limb of internal capsule and adjacent corona radiata
Pure sensory syndrome	Ventral posterior nucleus of thalamus

Anterior cerebral artery (ACA)

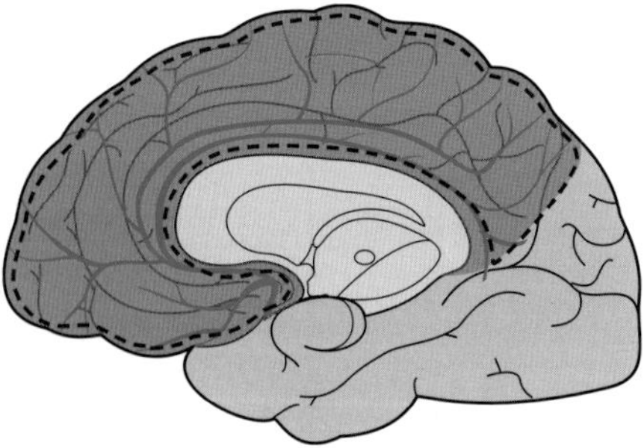

Figure 2.11 Anterior cerebral artery.

The anterior cerebral artery arises from the internal carotid artery and is connected by the anterior communicating artery.

It follows the curve of the corpus callosum and supplies the medial aspect of the frontal and parietal lobes, corpus callosum, internal capsule and basal ganglia (caudate nucleus and globus pallidus).

Signs and symptoms	Structures involved
Contralateral hemiplegia/hemiparesis (lower limb > upper limb)	Motor cortex
Contralateral sensory loss/ impairment (lower limb > upper limb)	Somatosensory cortex
Urinary incontinence	Superior frontal gyrus (bilateral)
Contralateral grasp reflex	Frontal lobe
Akinetic mutism, whispering, apathy	Frontal lobe (bilateral)
Apraxia of left limbs	Corpus callosum
Tactile agnosia	Corpus callosum
Spastic paresis of lower limb	Bilateral motor leg area

Posterior cerebral artery (PCA)

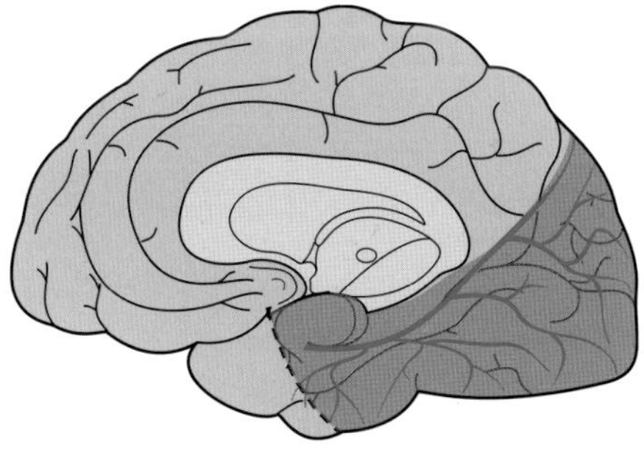

Figure 2.12 Posterior cerebral artery.

The posterior cerebral artery arises from the basilar artery. It supplies the occipital and temporal lobes, midbrain, choroid plexus, thalamus, subthalamic nucleus, optic radiation, corpus callosum and cranial nerves III and IV. The posterior communicating arteries connect the posterior cerebral arteries to the middle cerebral arteries anteriorly.

Signs and symptoms	Structures involved
Thalamic syndrome: hemisensory loss, chorea or hemiballism, spontaneous pain and dysaesthesias	Posterior nucleus of thalamus
Weber's syndrome: oculomotor paralysis and contralateral hemiplegia	Cranial nerve III and cerebral peduncle
Contralateral hemiballism	Subthalamic nucleus
Contralateral homonymous hemianopia	Primary visual cortex or optic radiation
Bilateral homonymous hemianopia, visual hallucinations	Bilateral occipital lobe
Alexia, colour anomia, impaired memory	Dominant corpus callosum (occipital lobe)
Memory defect, amnesia	Bilateral inferomedial portions of temporal lobe
Prosopagnosia	Calcarine sulcus and lingual gyrus (non-dominant occipital lobe)

Vertebral and basilar arteries

The vertebral arteries arise from the subclavian arteries at the root of the neck and enter the skull through the foramen magnum. Within the skull they fuse to form the basilar artery. They supply the medulla, pons, midbrain and cerebellum.

Signs and symptoms	Structures involved
Lateral medullary syndrome: – vertigo, vomiting, nystagmus – ipsilateral limb ataxia – ipsilateral loss of facial pain and thermal sensation – ipsilateral Horner's syndrome – ipsilateral dysphagia, hoarseness, vocal cord paralysis and reduced gag reflex – contralateral loss of pain and thermal sensation in trunk and limbs	 Vestibular nuclei Spinocerebellar tract Cranial nerve V Descending sympathetic tract Cranial nerves IX and X Lateral spinothalamic tract
Ipsilateral tongue paralysis and hemiatrophy	Cranial nerve XII
Contralateral impaired tactile sensation and proprioception	Medial lemniscus
Diplopia, lateral and vertical gaze palsies, pupillary abnormalities	Cranial nerve VI, medial longitudinal fasciculus
Bulbar palsy, tetraplegia, changes in consciousness	Bilateral corticospinal tracts
Pseudobulbar palsy, emotional instability	Bilateral supranuclear fibres, cranial nerves IX–XII
Locked-in syndrome	Bilateral medulla or pons
Coma, death	Brainstem

Signs and symptoms of injury to the lobes of the brain (Lindsay & Bone 1997, with permission)

Frontal lobe

Function	**Signs of impairment**
Precentral gyrus (motor cortex) Contralateral movement: face, arm, leg, trunk	Contralateral hemiparesis/ hemiplegia
Broca's area (dominant hemisphere) Expressive centre for speech	Broca's dysphasia (dominant)
Supplementary motor area Contralateral head and eye turning	Paralysis of contralateral head and eye movement
Prefrontal areas 'Personality', initiative	Disinhibition, poor judgement, akinesia, indifference, emotional lability, gait disturbance, incontinence, primitive reflexes, e.g. grasp
Paracentral lobule Cortical inhibition of bladder and bowel voiding	Incontinence of urine and faeces

Parietal lobe

Function	**Signs of impairment**
Postcentral gyrus (sensory cortex) Posture, touch and passive movement	Hemisensory loss/disturbance: postural, passive movement, localization of light touch, two-point discrimination, astereognosis, sensory inattention

Function	Signs of impairment
Supramarginal and angular gyri: *Dominant hemisphere (part of Wernicke's language area)* Integration of auditory and visual aspects of comprehension	Wernicke's dysphasia
Non-dominant hemisphere Body image, awareness of external environment, ability to construct shapes, etc.	Left-sided inattention, denies hemiparesis Anosognosia, dressing apraxia, geographical agnosia, constructional apraxia
Dominant parietal lobe Calculation, using numbers	Finger agnosia, acalculia, agraphia, confusion between right and left
Optic radiation Visual pathways	Homonymous quadrantanopia

Temporal lobe

Function	Signs of impairment
Superior temporal gyrus (auditory cortex) Hearing of language (dominant hemisphere), hearing of sounds, rhythm and music (non-dominant)	Cortical deafness, difficulty hearing speech – associated with Wernicke's dysphasia (dominant), amusia (non-dominant), auditory hallucinations
Middle and inferior temporal gyri Learning and memory	Disturbance of memory and learning
Limbic lobe Smell, emotional/affective behaviour	Olfactory hallucination, aggressive or antisocial behaviour, inability to establish new memories
Optic radiation Visual pathways	Upper homonymous quadrantanopia

Occipital lobe

Function	Signs of impairment
Calcarine sulcus *Primary visual/striate cortex* Relay of visual information to parastriate cortex	Cortical blindness (bilateral involvement), homonymous hemianopia with or without macular involvement
Association visual/parastriate cortex Relay of visual information to parietal, temporal and frontal lobes	Cortical blindness without awareness (striate and parastriate involvement), inability to direct gaze associated with agnosia (bilateral parieto-occipital lesions), prosopagnosia (bilateral occipito-temporal lesions)

Signs and symptoms of haemorrhage to other areas of the brain

Putamen

Function	Signs of impairment
Part of basal ganglia Involved in selective movement	Contralateral hemiplegia/hemiparesis, contralateral hemisensory loss, hemianopia (posterior segment), contralateral gaze palsy (posterior segment), Wernicke-type dysphasia (posterior segment, left side), anosognosia (posterior segment, right side), apathy, motor impersistence, temporary unilateral neglect (anterior segment), coma/death (large lesion)

Thalamus

Function	Signs of impairment
Thalamus Receives motor and sensory inputs and transmits them to the cerebral cortex	Contralateral hemiparesis/hemiplegia, contralateral hemisensory loss, impaired consciousness, ocular disturbances (varied), dysphasia (dominant), contralateral neglect (non-dominant)

Pons

Function	Signs of impairment
Part of brainstem Contains descending motor pathways, ascending sensory pathways and cranial nerve nuclei V–VIII	Coma/death (large bilateral lesions), locked-in syndrome (bilateral), tetraplegia (bilateral), lateral gaze palsy towards affected side, contralateral hemiplegia, contralateral hemisensory loss, ipsilateral facial weakness/ sensory loss

Cerebellum

Function	Signs of impairment
Anterior lobe (spinocerebellum) Muscle tone, posture and gait control	Hypotonia, postural reflex abnormalities
Posterior lobe (neocerebellum) Coordination of skilled movements	Ipsilateral ataxia: dysmetria, dysdiadochokinesia, intention tremor, rebound phenomenon, dyssynergia, dysarthria
Flocculonodular lobe (vestibulocerebellum) Eye movements and balance	Disturbance of balance, unsteadiness of gait and stance, truncal ataxia, nystagmus, ocular disturbances

SECTION 2

Cranial nerves

The cranial nerves form part of the peripheral nervous system and originate from the brain. Each nerve is named according to its function or appearance and is numbered using roman numerals from I to XII. The numbers roughly correspond to their position as they descend from just above the brainstem (I and II), through the midbrain (III and IV), pons (V–VII) and medulla (VIII–XII).

Name	Function	Abnormal signs
Olfactory (I)	Smell	Partial or total loss of smell Altered or increased sense of smell
Optic (II)	Sight	Visual fields defects, loss of visual acuity, colourblindness
Oculomotor (III)	Movement of eyelid and eyeball, constriction of pupil, lens accommodation	Squint, ptosis, diplopia, pupil dilation
Trochlear (IV)	Movement of eyeball upwards	Diplopia, squint
Trigeminal (V)	Mastication, sensation for eye, face, sinuses and teeth	Trigeminal neuralgia, loss of mastication and sensation in eye, face, sinuses and teeth
Abducens (VI)	Movement of eyeball into abduction, controls gaze	Gaze palsy
Facial (VII)	Facial movements, sensation and taste for anterior two-thirds of tongue, secretion of saliva and tears	Bell's palsy, loss of taste and ability to close eyes

Name	Function	Abnormal signs
Vestibulo-cochlear (VIII)	Hearing, balance	Tinnitus, deafness, vertigo, ataxia, nystagmus
Glosso-pharyngeal (IX)	Sensation and taste for posterior third of tongue, swallow, salivation, regulation of blood pressure	Loss of tongue sensation and taste, reduced salivation, dysphagia
Vagus (X)	Motor and sensation for heart, lungs, digestive tract and diaphragm, secretion of digestive fluids, taste, swallow, hiccups	Vocal cord paralysis, dysphagia, loss of sensation from internal organs
Accessory (XI)	Motor to soft palate, larynx, pharynx, trapezius and sternocleidomastoid	Paralysis of innervated muscles
Hypoglossal (XII)	Tongue control and strap muscles of neck	Dysphagia, dysarthria, difficulty masticating

Key features of upper and lower motor neurone lesions

	Upper motor neurone	Lower motor neurone
Muscle tone	Increased	Decreased
Clonus	Present	Absent
Muscle fasciculation	Absent	Present
Tendon reflexes	Increased	Depressed or absent
Plantar response	Extensor (Babinski's sign)	Flexor (normal)

	Upper motor neurone	Lower motor neurone
Distribution	Extensor weakness in upper limb and flexor weakness in lower limb. Whole limb(s) involved	Weakness of muscle groups innervated by affected spinal segment/root, plexus or peripheral nerve

Upper motor neurone

Origin: cerebral cortex
Terminates: cranial nerve nuclei or spinal cord anterior horn

Lower motor neurone

Origin: cranial nerve motor nuclei or spinal cord anterior horn
Terminates: skeletal muscle motor unit

Muscle innervation chart (data from Williams 1995, with permission)

Upper limb

<table>
<tr><th>C1</th><th>C2</th><th>C3</th><th>C4</th><th>C5</th><th>C6</th><th>C7</th><th>C8</th><th>T1</th></tr>
<tr><td>Inferior and superior oblique</td><td></td><td></td><td></td><td></td><td></td><td></td><td></td><td></td></tr>
<tr><td>Rectus capitis posterior major and minor</td><td></td><td></td><td></td><td></td><td></td><td></td><td></td><td></td></tr>
<tr><td colspan="2">Rectus capitis anterior and lateralis</td><td></td><td></td><td></td><td></td><td></td><td></td><td></td></tr>
<tr><td colspan="3">Longus capitis</td><td></td><td></td><td></td><td></td><td></td><td></td></tr>
</table>

<table>
<tr><th>C1</th><th>C2</th><th>C3</th><th>C4</th><th>C5</th><th>C6</th><th>C7</th><th>C8</th><th>T1</th></tr>
<tr><td></td><td colspan="5">Longissimus cervicis</td><td></td><td></td><td></td></tr>
<tr><td></td><td colspan="5">Longus colli</td><td></td><td></td><td></td></tr>
<tr><td></td><td></td><td colspan="2">Levator scapulae</td><td></td><td></td><td></td><td></td><td></td></tr>
<tr><td></td><td></td><td colspan="2">Trapezius</td><td></td><td></td><td></td><td></td><td></td></tr>
<tr><td></td><td></td><td colspan="3">Diaphragm</td><td></td><td></td><td></td><td></td></tr>
<tr><td></td><td></td><td colspan="3">Splenius capitis</td><td></td><td></td><td></td><td></td></tr>
<tr><td></td><td></td><td colspan="6">Scalenus medius</td><td></td></tr>
<tr><td></td><td></td><td></td><td colspan="2">Rhomboid major</td><td></td><td></td><td></td><td></td></tr>
<tr><td></td><td></td><td></td><td colspan="2">Rhomboid minor</td><td></td><td></td><td></td><td></td></tr>
<tr><td></td><td></td><td></td><td colspan="3">Scalenus anterior</td><td></td><td></td><td></td></tr>
<tr><td></td><td></td><td></td><td colspan="4">Longissimus capitis</td><td></td><td></td></tr>
<tr><td></td><td></td><td></td><td></td><td colspan="2">Biceps brachii</td><td></td><td></td><td></td></tr>
<tr><td></td><td></td><td></td><td></td><td colspan="2">Brachioradialis</td><td></td><td></td><td></td></tr>
<tr><td></td><td></td><td></td><td></td><td colspan="2">Deltoid</td><td></td><td></td><td></td></tr>
<tr><td></td><td></td><td></td><td></td><td colspan="2">Infraspinatus</td><td></td><td></td><td></td></tr>
<tr><td></td><td></td><td></td><td></td><td colspan="2">Subscapularis</td><td></td><td></td><td></td></tr>
<tr><td></td><td></td><td></td><td></td><td colspan="2">Supraspinatus</td><td></td><td></td><td></td></tr>
<tr><td></td><td></td><td></td><td></td><td colspan="2">Teres minor</td><td></td><td></td><td></td></tr>
<tr><td></td><td></td><td></td><td></td><td colspan="3">Brachialis</td><td></td><td></td></tr>
<tr><td></td><td></td><td></td><td></td><td colspan="3">Coracobrachialis</td><td></td><td></td></tr>
<tr><td></td><td></td><td></td><td></td><td colspan="3">Serratus anterior</td><td></td><td></td></tr>
<tr><td></td><td></td><td></td><td></td><td colspan="3">Splenius cervicis</td><td></td><td></td></tr>
<tr><td></td><td></td><td></td><td></td><td colspan="3">Teres major</td><td></td><td></td></tr>
<tr><td></td><td></td><td></td><td></td><td colspan="5">Pectoralis major</td></tr>
<tr><td></td><td></td><td></td><td></td><td colspan="5">Pectoralis minor</td></tr>
<tr><td></td><td></td><td></td><td></td><td></td><td colspan="2">Extensor carpi radialis longus</td><td></td><td></td></tr>
<tr><td></td><td></td><td></td><td></td><td></td><td colspan="2">Flexor carpi radialis</td><td></td><td></td></tr>
<tr><td></td><td></td><td></td><td></td><td></td><td colspan="2">Pronator teres</td><td></td><td></td></tr>
<tr><td></td><td></td><td></td><td></td><td></td><td colspan="2">Supinator</td><td></td><td></td></tr>
<tr><td></td><td></td><td></td><td></td><td></td><td colspan="3">Anconeus</td><td></td></tr>
<tr><td></td><td></td><td></td><td></td><td></td><td colspan="3">Latissimus dorsi</td><td></td></tr>
<tr><td></td><td></td><td></td><td></td><td></td><td colspan="3">Scalenus posterior</td><td></td></tr>
<tr><td></td><td></td><td></td><td></td><td></td><td colspan="3">Triceps brachii</td><td></td></tr>
</table>

C1	C2	C3	C4	C5	C6	C7	C8	T1
						Abductor pollicis longus		
						Extensor carpi radialis brevis		
						Extensor carpi ulnaris		
						Extensor digiti minimi		
						Extensor digitorum		
						Extensor indicis		
						Extensor pollicis brevis		
						Extensor pollicis longus		
						Flexor pollicis longus		
						Palmaris longus		
						Pronator quadratus		
						Flexor carpi ulnaris		
							Abductor digiti minimi	
							Abductor pollicis brevis	
							Adductor pollicis	
							Dorsal interossei	
							Flexor digiti minimi brevis	
							Flexor digitorum profundus	
							Flexor digitorum superficialis	
							Flexor pollicis brevis	
							Lumbricals	
							Opponens digiti minimi	
							Opponens pollicis	
							Palmar interossei	

Lower limb

<table>
<tr><th>T12</th><th>L1</th><th>L2</th><th>L3</th><th>L4</th><th>L5</th><th>S1</th><th>S2</th><th>S3</th></tr>
<tr><td colspan="5">Quadratus lumborum</td><td></td><td></td><td></td><td></td></tr>
<tr><td></td><td>Psoas minor</td><td></td><td></td><td></td><td></td><td></td><td></td><td></td></tr>
<tr><td></td><td colspan="3">Psoas major</td><td></td><td></td><td></td><td></td><td></td></tr>
<tr><td></td><td></td><td colspan="2">Adductor brevis</td><td></td><td></td><td></td><td></td><td></td></tr>
<tr><td></td><td></td><td colspan="2">Gracilis</td><td></td><td></td><td></td><td></td><td></td></tr>
<tr><td></td><td></td><td colspan="2">Iliacus</td><td></td><td></td><td></td><td></td><td></td></tr>
<tr><td></td><td></td><td colspan="2">Pectineus</td><td></td><td></td><td></td><td></td><td></td></tr>
<tr><td></td><td></td><td colspan="2">Sartorius</td><td></td><td></td><td></td><td></td><td></td></tr>
<tr><td></td><td></td><td colspan="3">Adductor longus</td><td></td><td></td><td></td><td></td></tr>
<tr><td></td><td></td><td colspan="3">Adductor magnus</td><td></td><td></td><td></td><td></td></tr>
<tr><td></td><td></td><td colspan="3">Rectus femoris</td><td></td><td></td><td></td><td></td></tr>
<tr><td></td><td></td><td colspan="3">Vastus intermedius</td><td></td><td></td><td></td><td></td></tr>
<tr><td></td><td></td><td colspan="3">Vastus lateralis</td><td></td><td></td><td></td><td></td></tr>
<tr><td></td><td></td><td colspan="3">Vastus medialis</td><td></td><td></td><td></td><td></td></tr>
<tr><td></td><td></td><td></td><td colspan="2">Obturator externus</td><td></td><td></td><td></td><td></td></tr>
<tr><td></td><td></td><td></td><td colspan="3">Gluteus medius</td><td></td><td></td><td></td></tr>
<tr><td></td><td></td><td></td><td colspan="3">Gluteus minimus</td><td></td><td></td><td></td></tr>
<tr><td></td><td></td><td></td><td colspan="3">Popliteus</td><td></td><td></td><td></td></tr>
<tr><td></td><td></td><td></td><td></td><td colspan="2">Tibialis anterior</td><td></td><td></td><td></td></tr>
<tr><td></td><td></td><td></td><td></td><td colspan="2">Tibialis posterior</td><td></td><td></td><td></td></tr>
<tr><td></td><td></td><td></td><td></td><td colspan="3">Tensor fascia lata</td><td></td><td></td></tr>
<tr><td></td><td></td><td></td><td></td><td></td><td>Extensor hallucis longus</td><td></td><td></td><td></td></tr>
<tr><td></td><td></td><td></td><td></td><td></td><td colspan="2">Extensor digitorum brevis</td><td></td><td></td></tr>
<tr><td></td><td></td><td></td><td></td><td></td><td colspan="2">Extensor digitorum longus</td><td></td><td></td></tr>
<tr><td></td><td></td><td></td><td></td><td></td><td colspan="2">Gemellus inferior</td><td></td><td></td></tr>
<tr><td></td><td></td><td></td><td></td><td></td><td colspan="2">Gemellus superior</td><td></td><td></td></tr>
<tr><td></td><td></td><td></td><td></td><td></td><td colspan="2">Obturator internus</td><td></td><td></td></tr>
</table>

<table>
<tr><th>T12</th><th>L1</th><th>L2</th><th>L3</th><th>L4</th><th>L5</th><th>S1</th><th>S2</th><th>S3</th></tr>
<tr><td></td><td></td><td></td><td></td><td></td><td colspan="2">Peroneus brevis</td><td></td><td></td></tr>
<tr><td></td><td></td><td></td><td></td><td></td><td colspan="2">Peroneus longus</td><td></td><td></td></tr>
<tr><td></td><td></td><td></td><td></td><td></td><td colspan="2">Peroneus tertius</td><td></td><td></td></tr>
<tr><td></td><td></td><td></td><td></td><td></td><td colspan="2">Quadratus femoris</td><td></td><td></td></tr>
<tr><td></td><td></td><td></td><td></td><td></td><td colspan="3">Biceps femoris</td><td></td></tr>
<tr><td></td><td></td><td></td><td></td><td></td><td colspan="3">Flexor digitorum longus</td><td></td></tr>
<tr><td></td><td></td><td></td><td></td><td></td><td colspan="3">Flexor hallucis longus</td><td></td></tr>
<tr><td></td><td></td><td></td><td></td><td></td><td colspan="3">Gluteus maximus</td><td></td></tr>
<tr><td></td><td></td><td></td><td></td><td></td><td colspan="3">Piriformis</td><td></td></tr>
<tr><td></td><td></td><td></td><td></td><td></td><td colspan="3">Semimembranosus</td><td></td></tr>
<tr><td></td><td></td><td></td><td></td><td></td><td colspan="3">Semitendinosus</td><td></td></tr>
<tr><td></td><td></td><td></td><td></td><td></td><td></td><td colspan="2">Abductor hallucis</td><td></td></tr>
<tr><td></td><td></td><td></td><td></td><td></td><td></td><td colspan="2">Flexor digitorum brevis</td><td></td></tr>
<tr><td></td><td></td><td></td><td></td><td></td><td></td><td colspan="2">Flexor hallucis brevis</td><td></td></tr>
<tr><td></td><td></td><td></td><td></td><td></td><td></td><td colspan="2">Gastrocnemius</td><td></td></tr>
<tr><td></td><td></td><td></td><td></td><td></td><td></td><td colspan="2">Plantaris</td><td></td></tr>
<tr><td></td><td></td><td></td><td></td><td></td><td></td><td colspan="2">Soleus</td><td></td></tr>
<tr><td></td><td></td><td></td><td></td><td></td><td></td><td colspan="3">Abductor digiti minimi</td></tr>
<tr><td></td><td></td><td></td><td></td><td></td><td></td><td colspan="3">Flexor digitorum accessorius</td></tr>
<tr><td></td><td></td><td></td><td></td><td></td><td></td><td></td><td colspan="2">Adductor hallucis</td></tr>
<tr><td></td><td></td><td></td><td></td><td></td><td></td><td></td><td colspan="2">Dorsal interossei</td></tr>
<tr><td></td><td></td><td></td><td></td><td></td><td></td><td></td><td colspan="2">Flexor digiti minimi brevis</td></tr>
<tr><td></td><td></td><td></td><td></td><td></td><td></td><td></td><td colspan="2">Lumbricals</td></tr>
<tr><td></td><td></td><td></td><td></td><td></td><td></td><td></td><td colspan="2">Plantar interossei</td></tr>
</table>

Functional implications of spinal cord injury

Level	Motor control	Personal independence	Equipment	Mobility
C1–C2	Swallow, talk, chew, blow (cough absent)	Type, turn pages, use telephone and computer	Hoist, respirator, mouthstick, reclining powered wheelchair using breath/chin control	Wheelchair
C3	Neck control, weak shoulder elevation	As above	Hoist, respirator, mouth/head stick, wheelchair as above	Wheelchair
C4	Respiration, neck control, shoulder shrug	Feed possible	Mouth/head stick, hoist, mobile arm supports, wheelchair as above	Wheelchair
C5	Shoulder external rotation, protraction, elbow flexion, supination	Feed, groom, roll in bed, weight shift, push wheelchair on flat, use brake	Adapted feeding/ grooming equipment and hand splints, mobile arm supports, powered wheelchair with hand controls or lightweight manual with grips	Wheelchair

Level	Motor control	Personal independence	Equipment	Mobility
C6	Shoulder, elbow flexion, wrist extension, pronation. Weak elbow extension, wrist flexion and thumb control	Tenodesis grip, drink, write, personal ADL, transfers, dress upper body, light domestic chores, push wheelchair on slope	Adapted equipment and splints, transfer board, hand controlled car, lightweight manual wheelchair, powered for short distances	Bed mobility, bed to chair transfers, wheelchair, car
C7	Elbow extension, finger flexion and extension, limited wrist flexion	Dress lower body, personal and skin care, showering, all transfers, pick up from floor, wheelchair sports	Bath board, shower chair, hand controlled car, wheelchair as above	All transfers, wheelchair, car
C8	Wrist flexion, hand control	Bladder and bowel care	Grab rails, standing frame, non-adapted wheelchair	Stand in frame
T1–T5	Top half of intercostals and long back muscles	Trunk support, improved balance, assisted cough, negotiate kerbs	Bilateral knee–ankle orthoses with spinal attachment, standing frame/table	Full wheelchair independence, transfer floor to chair,

		with wheelchair, routine domestic chores		mobilize with assistance for short distances
T6–T12	Abdominals	Good balance, weak to normal cough, improved stamina	Bilateral knee–ankle orthoses, crutches or frame	Mobilize independently indoors, transfer chair to crutches
L1–L2	Hip flexion		Calipers	Stairs, transfer floor to crutches
L3–L5	Knee extension, weak knee flexion, dorsiflexion and eversion		Ankle–foot orthoses, crutches/sticks	
S1–S2	Hip extension	Improved standing balance		Normal gait without aids
S2–S4	Bladder, bowel and sexual function			

Neurological pathologies

Alzheimer's disease

A form of dementia that is characterized by slow, progressive mental deterioration. Symptoms may start with mild forgetfulness, difficulty remembering names and faces or recent events and progress to memory failure, disorientation, speech disturbances, motor impairment and aggressive behaviour. It is the most common form of dementia and is distinguished by the presence of neuritic plaques (primarily in the hippocampus and parietal lobes), and neurofibrillary tangles (mainly affecting the pyramidal cells of the cortex). Definitive diagnosis is post-mortem.

Bell's palsy

An acute, lower motor neurone paralysis of the face, usually unilateral, related to inflammation and swelling of the facial nerve (VII) within the facial canal or at the stylomastoid foramen. Symptoms include inability to close the eye on the affected side, hyperacusis and impairment of taste. Good recovery is common.

Broca's dysphasia

A lesion of Broca's area, on the inferior frontal cortex, causing non-fluent, hesitant speech that is characterized by poor grammar and reduced word output while meaning is preserved. Perseverance can occur and writing may be impaired but comprehension remains relatively intact. Broca's area is near the motor cortex for the face and arm and so may be associated with weakness in these areas.

Brown-Sequard syndrome

A neurological condition that occurs when there is damage to one half of the spinal cord. Below the lesion there is motor loss on the same side and loss of pain and temperature on the opposite side.

Bulbar palsy

A bilateral or unilateral lower motor neurone lesion that affects the nerves supplying the bulbar muscles of the head and neck. Causes paralysis or weakness of the muscles of the jaw, face, palate, pharynx and larynx leading to impaired swallow, cough, gag reflex and speech.

Cerebral palsy

An umbrella term for a variety of posture and movement disorders arising from permanent brain damage incurred before, during, or immediately after birth. The disorder is most frequently associated with premature births and is often complicated by other neurological problems including epilepsy, visual, hearing and sensory impairments, communication and feeding difficulties, cognitive and behavioural problems. Common causes include intrauterine infection, intrauterine cerebrovascular insult, birth asphyxia, postnatal meningitis and postnatal cerebrovascular insult. The most common disability is a spastic paralysis, which can be associated with choreoathetosis (irregular, repetitive, writhing and jerky movements).

Charcot–Marie–Tooth disease

A progressive hereditary disorder of the peripheral nerves that is characterized by gradual progressive distal weakness and wasting, mainly affecting the peroneal muscle in the leg. Early symptoms include difficulty running and foot deformities. The disease is slowly progressive and in the late stages the arm muscles can also be involved. Also known as hereditary motor sensory neuropathy (HMSN).

Guillain–Barré syndrome (GBS)

An acute inflammatory polyneuropathy that usually occurs 1–4 weeks after fever associated with viral infection or following immunization. Thought to be an autoimmune disorder it leads to segmental demyelination of spinal roots and axons, denervation atrophy of muscle and inflammatory infiltration of the brain, liver, kidneys and lungs. Clinical features include loss of sensation in hands and feet, symmetrical progressive ascending motor weakness, paralysis, muscle wasting, diminished reflexes, pain and autonomic disturbances. In severe cases, the respiratory and bulbar systems are affected and ventilation/tracheostomy may be required. Recovery is common.

Horner's syndrome

A group of symptoms caused by a lesion of the sympathetic pathways in the hypothalamus, brainstem, spinal cord, C8–T2 ventral spinal roots, superior cervical ganglion or internal carotid sheath. It causes ipsilateral pupil constriction, drooping of the upper eyelid and loss of facial sweating on the affected side of the face.

Huntingdon's disease

A hereditary disease caused by a defect in chromosome 4 that can be inherited from either parent. Onset is insidious and occurs between 35 and 50 years of age. Symptoms include sudden, involuntary movements (chorea) accompanied by behavioural changes and progressive dementia.

Locked-in syndrome

A rare neurological disorder characterized by total paralysis of all voluntary muscles except those controlling eye movement and some facial movements. May be caused by traumatic brain injury, vascular disease, demyelinating diseases or overdose. Patients are unable to speak or move but sight, hearing and cognition are normal. Prognosis for recovery is poor with most patients not regaining function.

Meningitis

An acute inflammation of the meninges due to infection by bacteria or viruses. Age groups most at risk are the under 5s, especially infants under the age of 1 year, and adolescents between 15 and 19 years of age. The most common causes of bacterial meningitis in young children are *Neisseria meningitidis* (meningococcal meningitis) and *Haemophilus influenzae.* The classic triad of clinical features is fever, headache and neck stiffness. Skin rash and septic shock may occur where septicaemia has developed as a result of widespread meningococcal infection. Other signs in adults include confusion and photophobia. Onset of symptoms may be gradual or sudden; however, deterioration is rapid, often requiring intensive supportive therapy.

Motor neurone disease

A group of progressive degenerative diseases of the motor system occurring in middle to late adult life, causing weakness, wasting and eventual paralysis of muscles. It primarily affects the anterior horn cells of the spinal cord, the motor nuclei of the brainstem and the corticospinal tracts. There are three distinct types:

Progressive muscle atrophy

Starts early in life, typically before 50 years of age. Affects cervical region leading to atrophy of the muscles of the hand. Involvement spreads to the arms and shoulder girdle and may extend to the legs.

Amyotrophic lateral sclerosis

There are upper motor neurone changes as well as lower motor neurone changes. Characterized by weakness and atrophy in the hands, forearms and legs but may also spread to the body and face.

Progressive bulbar palsy

Caused by damage to the motor nuclei in the bulbar region in the brainstem which results in wasting and paralysis of muscles of the mouth, jaw, larynx and pharynx. General features include pain and spasms, dyspnoea, dysphagia, dysarthria and sore eyes.

Multiple sclerosis

A chronic, progressive disease characterized by multiple demyelinating lesions (plaques) throughout the central nervous system. It predominantly affects young adults in temperate latitudes and is more prevalent in women. The disease is usually characterized by recurrent relapses (attacks) followed by remissions, although some patients follow a chronic, progressive course. The plaques interfere with normal nerve impulses along the nerve fibre and the site of the lesions and the degree of inflammation at each site leads to a variety of neurological signs and symptoms. Common symptoms include visual disturbances, ataxia, sensory and motor disturbance, bulbar dysfunction, fatigue, bladder and bowel symptoms, cognitive and emotional disturbances, pain and spasm.

Muscular dystrophy

A group of genetically determined progressive muscle wasting diseases in which the affected muscle fibres degenerate and are replaced by fat and connective tissue. Duchenne muscular dystrophy is the most common form, affecting boys before the age of 4 years. Clinical features include difficulty walking, pseudohypertrophy of proximal muscles, postural problems, diminished reflexes and difficulty standing from squatting (Gower's sign).

Myasthenia gravis

A disorder of the neuromuscular junction caused by an impaired ability of the neurotransmitter acetylcholine to induce muscular contraction, most likely due to an autoimmune destruction of the postsynaptic receptors for acetylcholine. It predominantly affects adolescents and young adults (mainly women) and is characterized by abnormal weakness and fatiguing of some or all muscle groups to the point of temporary paralysis. Onset of symptoms is usually gradual and includes drooping of the upper eyelid, double vision, dysarthria and weakness of other facial muscles.

Parkinson's disease

A degenerative disease of the substantia nigra that reduces the amount of dopamine in the basal ganglia. Depletion of dopamine levels affects the ability of the basal ganglia to control movement, posture and coordination and leads to the characteristic symptoms of rigidity, slowness of voluntary movement, poor postural reflexes and resting tremor. Parkinson's has a gradual, insidious onset and affects mainly those aged between 50 and 65 years. Early symptoms of Parkinson's include aches and stiffness, difficulty with fine manipulative movements, slowness of walking, resting tremor of head, hands (pill rolling) and feet while later symptoms may include shuffling gait, difficulties with speech, a mask-like appearance and depression.

Poliomyelitis

Poliomyelitis is a highly contagious infectious disease caused by one of three types of poliovirus. The extent of the disease varies, with some people experiencing no or mild symptoms, while others develop the paralytic form of the disease. It can strike at any age, but affects mainly children under the age of 3. The poliovirus destroys motor neurones in the anterior horn. The muscles of the legs are affected more often than those of the arm but the paralysis can spread to the muscles of the thorax and abdomen. In the most severe form (bulbar polio), the motor neurones of the brainstem are attacked, reducing breathing capacity and causing difficulty in swallowing and speaking. Without respiratory support, bulbar polio can result in death.

Post polio syndrome

A recurrence or progression of neuromuscular symptoms that appears in people who have recovered from acute paralytic poliomyelitis, usually 15–40 years after the original illness. Symptoms include progressive muscle weakness, severe fatigue and pain in muscles and joints.

Pseudobulbar palsy

An upper motor neurone lesion that affects the corticomotor-neurone pathways and results in weakness and spasticity of the oral and pharyngeal musculature. Leads to slurring of speech and dysphagia. Patients also exhibit emotional incontinence. They are unable to control their emotional expression and may laugh or cry without apparent reason.

Spinal muscular atrophies (SMA)

A group of inherited degenerative disorders of the anterior horn cell causing muscle atrophy. There are three main types, which are classified by age of onset: *SMA I (Werdnig–Hoffman disease)* is the most severe form with onset from preterm to 6 months. It causes weakness and hypotonia ('floppy' babies) leading to death within 3 years. *SMA II (intermediate type)* usually develops between 6 and 15 months of age. It has the same pathological features as SMA I but progresses more slowly. *SMA III (Wohlfart–Kugelberg–Welander disease)* has a late onset, between 1 year and adolescence, leading to progressive, proximal limb weakness.

Stroke/cerebrovascular accident (CVA)

An illness in which part of the brain is suddenly severely damaged or destroyed as a consequence of an interruption to the flow of blood in the brain. This interruption may be caused by a blood clot (ischaemic stroke) or by a ruptured blood vessel (haemorrhagic stroke), either within the brain (intracerebral) or around the brain (subarachnoid). The most common symptoms of stroke are numbness, weakness or paralysis on one side of the body, contralateral to the side of the brain in which the cerebrovascular accident occurred. Other symptoms include dysphasia, dysphagia, dysarthria, dyspraxia, disturbance of vision and perception, inattention or unilateral neglect, and memory or attention problems. Where symptoms resolve within 24 hours, this is known as a transient ischaemic attack (TIA).

Transverse myelitis

A demyelinating disorder of the spinal cord where inflammation spreads more or less completely across the tissue of the spinal cord resulting in a loss of its normal function to transmit nerve impulses up and down. Paralysis and numbness affect the legs and trunk below the level of diseased tissue. Causes include spinal cord injury, immune reaction, atherosclerotic vascular disease and viral infection, e.g. smallpox, measles, or chickenpox. Some patients progress to multiple sclerosis. Recovery varies.

Trigeminal neuralgia

A condition that is characterized by brief attacks of severe, sharp, stabbing facial pain in the territory of one or more divisions of the trigeminal nerve (cranial nerve V). It can be caused by degeneration of the nerve or compression on it (e.g. by a tumour), though often the cause is unknown. Attacks can last for several days or weeks after which the patient may be pain-free for months.

Wernicke's dysphasia

A lesion of Wernicke's area (posterolateral left temporal and inferior parietal language region of the left cortex) causing fluent but nonsensical speech. Writing and comprehension are greatly impaired. The patient is unaware of the language problem.

Glossary of neurological terms

Acalculia	inability to calculate
Agnosia	inability to interpret sensations such as sounds (auditory agnosia), three-dimensional objects by touch (tactile agnosia) or symbols and letters (visual agnosia)
Agraphia	inability to write
Akinesia	loss of movement
Alexia	inability to read
Amnesia	total or partial loss of memory
Amusia	impaired recognition of music
Anomia	inability to name objects
Anosmia	loss of ability to smell
Anosognosia	denial of ownership or the existence of a hemiplegic limb
Aphasia	inability to generate and understand language whether verbal or written
Astereognosis	inability to recognize objects by touch alone, despite intact sensation
Ataxia	shaky and uncoordinated voluntary movements that may be associated with cerebellar or posterior column disease
Athetosis	involuntary writhing movements affecting face, tongue and hands
Bradykinesia	slowness of movement
Chorea	irregular, jerky, involuntary movement
Clonus	more than three rhythmic contractions of the plantarflexors in response to sudden passive dorsiflexion
Diplopia	double vision

Dysaesthesia	perverted response to sensory stimuli producing abnormal and sometimes unpleasant sensation
Dysarthria	difficulty articulating speech
Dysdiadochokinesia	clumsiness in performing rapidly alternating movements
Dysmetria	under- or overshooting while reaching towards a target
Dysphagia	difficulty or inability to swallow
Dysphasia	difficulty understanding language (receptive dysphasia) or generating language (expressive dysphasia)
Dysphonia	difficulty in producing the voice
Dyspraxia	inability to make skilled movements despite intact power, sensation and coordination
Dyssynergia	clumsy, uncoordinated movements
Dystonia	abnormal postural movements caused by co-contraction of agonists and antagonists, usually at an extreme of flexion or extension
Graphanaesthesia	inability to recognize numbers or letters traced onto the skin with a blunt object
Hemianopia	loss of half the normal visual field
Hemiballismus	sudden, involuntary violent flinging movements of an entire limb, usually unilateral
Hemiparesis	weakness affecting one side of the body
Hemiplegia	paralysis affecting one side of the body
Homonymous	affecting the same side, i.e. homonymous diplopia
Hyperacusis	increased sensitivity to sound
Hyperreflexia	increased reflexes

Hypertonia	increase in normal muscle tone
Hypertrophy	abnormal increase in tissue size
Kinaesthesia	perception of body position and movement
Miosis	pupil constriction
Nystagmus	involuntary movements of the eye
Paraesthesia	tingling sensation often described as 'pins and needles'
Paraphasia	insertion of inappropriate or incorrect words in person's speech
Paraplegia	paralysis of both legs
Paresis	muscle weakness
Photophobia	intolerance to light
Prosopagnosia	inability to recognize faces
Ptosis	drooping of the upper eyelid
Quadrantanopia	loss of quarter the normal visual field
Quadriplegia	paralysis of all four limbs
Stereognosis	ability to identify common objects by touch alone
Tetraplegia	another term for quadriplegia

Neurological assessment (based on ACPIN 1995, with permission)

Patients present with a variety of conditions and assessments need to be adapted to suit their needs. This chapter provides a basic framework for the subjective and objective neurological assessment of a patient.

Database

History of present condition
Past medical history
Drug history
Results of specific investigations (X-rays, CT scans, blood tests, etc.)

Subjective examination

Social situation
- family support
- accommodation
- employment
- leisure activities
- social service support

Normal daily routine
Indoor and outdoor mobility
Continence
Vision
Hearing
Swallowing
Fatigue
Pain
Other ongoing treatment
Past physiotherapy and response to treatment
Perceptions of own problems/main concern
Expectations of treatment

Objective examination

Posture and balance

Alignment
Neglect
Sitting balance
Standing balance
- Romberg test

Voluntary movement

Range of movement
Strength
Coordination
- finger to nose test
- heel to shin test
- rapidly alternating movement

Endurance

Involuntary movement
Tremor
Clonus
Chorea
Associated reactions

Tone
Decreased/flaccid
Increased
- spasticity (clasp-knife)
- rigidity (cogwheel or lead-pipe)

Reflexes
Deep tendon reflexes
- biceps (C5/6)
- triceps (C7/8)
- knee (L3/4)
- ankle (S1/2)

Plantar response (Babinski's sign)

Muscle and joint range
Passive range of movement

Sensory
Light touch
Pin prick
Two point discrimination
Vibration sense
Joint position sense
Temperature
Vision and hearing

Functional activities
Bed mobility
Sitting balance
Transfers
Upper limb function
Mobility
Stairs

Gait
Pattern
Distance
Velocity
Use of walking aids
Orthoses
Assistance from others

Exercise tolerance/fatigue

Cognitive status
Attention
Orientation
Memory

Emotional state

Neurological tests

Finger–nose test

Hold your finger about an arm's length from the patient. Ask the patient to touch your finger with their index finger and then touch their nose, repeating the movement back and forth. Patients may demonstrate past pointing (missing your finger) or intention tremor.
Indicates: possible cerebellar dysfunction.

Heel–shin test

With the patient lying down, ask them to place one heel on the opposite knee and then run the heel down the tibial shaft towards the ankle and back again. Patients may demonstrate intention tremor, an inability to keep the heel on the shin or uncoordinated movements.
Indicates: possible cerebellar dysfunction.

Joint position sense

Test the most distal joint of the limb, i.e. distal phalanx of the index finger or interphalangeal joint of the hallux. With the

patient's eyes open, demonstrate the movement. To test, get the patient to close their eyes. Hold the joint to be tested at the sides between two fingers and move it up and down. Ask the patient to identify the direction of movement, ensuring that you are not moving more proximal joints or brushing against the neighbouring toes or fingers. If there is impairment, test more proximal joints.
Indicates: loss of proprioception.

Light touch

Use a wisp of cotton wool. With the patient's eyes open, demonstrate what you are going to do. To test, get the patient to close their eyes. Stroke the patient's skin with the cotton wool at random points, asking them to indicate every time they feel the touch.
Indicates: altered touch sensation.

Pin prick

Use a disposable neurological pin which has a sharp end and a blunt end. With the patient's eyes open, demonstrate what you are going to do. To test, get the patient to close their eyes. Test various areas of the limb randomly using sharp and blunt stimuli and get the patient to tell you which sensation they feel.
Indicates: altered pain sensation.

Plantar response (Babinski)

Apply a firm pressure along the lateral aspect of the sole of the foot and across the base of the toes, observing the big toe. If the big toe flexes, the response is normal. If the big toe extends and the other toes spread it indicates a positive Babinski's sign.
Indicates: A positive Babinski's sign signifies an upper motor neurone lesion.

Rapidly alternating movement

Ask the patient to hold out one hand palm up and then alternately slap it with the palmar and then dorsal aspect of the

fingers of the other hand. Where there is a loss of rhythm and fluency it is referred to as dysdiadochokinesia. For the lower limbs get the patient to tap first one foot on the floor and then the other.
Indicates: possible cerebellar dysfunction.

Romberg's test

Patient stands with feet together and eyes open. Ask the patient to close their eyes (ensuring that you can support them if they fall). Note any excessive postural sway or loss of balance.
Indicates: proprioceptive or vestibular deficit if they fall only when they close their eyes.

Temperature

A quick test involves using a cold object such as a tuning fork and asking the patient to describe the sensation when applied to various parts of the body. For more formal testing, two test tubes are filled with cold and warm water and patients are asked to distinguish between the two sensations.
Indicates: altered temperature sensation.

Two-point discrimination

Requires a two-point discriminator, a device similar to a pair of blunted compasses. With the patient's eyes open, demonstrate what you are going to do. Get the patient to close their eyes. Alternately touch the patient with either one prong or two. Reduce the distance between the prongs until the patient can no longer discriminate between being touched by one prong or two prongs. Varies according to skin thickness but normal young patients can distinguish a separation of approximately 5 mm in the index finger and approximately 4 cm in the legs. Compare left to right.
Indicates: impaired sensory function.

SECTION 2

Vibration sense

Use a 128 Hz tuning fork. Ask the patient to close their eyes. Place the tuning fork on a bony prominence or on the fingertips or toes. The patient should report feeling the vibration and not simply the contact of the tuning fork. If in doubt, apply the tuning fork and then stop it vibrating suddenly by pinching it between your fingers and see if the patient can correctly identify when it stops vibrating.
Indicates: altered vibration sense.

References and further reading

ACPIN 1995 Neurological assessment. Standards of Physiotherapy Practice in Neurology. Association of Chartered Physiotherapists Interested in Neurology. Chartered Society of Physiotherapy. London

Association of Chartered Physiotherapists Interested in Neurology 1995 Standards of physiotherapy practice in neurology. ACPIN

Berlit P 1996 Memorix neurology. Chapman and Hall Medical, London

Bromley I 1998 Tetraplegia and paraplegia: a guide for physiotherapists, 5th edn. Churchill Livingstone, Edinburgh

Davies P M 2000 Steps to follow: the comprehensive treatment of patients with hemiplegia. Springer Verlag, Berlin

Fitzgerald M J T, Folan-Curran J 2002 Clinical neuroanatomy and related neuroscience, 4th edn. W B Saunders, Edinburgh

Fuller G 1999 Neurological examination made easy, 2nd edn. Churchill Livingstone, Edinburgh

Lasserson D, Gabriel C, Sharrack B 1998 Crash course: nervous system and special senses. Mosby, London

Lindsay K W, Bone I 1997 Neurology and neurosurgery illustrated, 3rd edn. Churchill Livingstone, New York

Marsden C D, Fowler T J 1998 Clinical neurology, 2nd edn. Arnold, London

Munro J, Edwards C 1995 Macleod's clinical examination, 9th edn. Churchill Livingstone, Edinburgh

Stokes M 1998 Neurological physiotherapy. Mosby, London

Victor M, Ropper A H 2001 Adams and Victor's principles of neurology, 7th edn. McGraw-Hill, New York

Williams P L 1995 Gray's anatomy, 38th edn. Churchill Livingstone, Edinburgh

SECTION 3

Respiratory

Respiratory anatomy illustrations

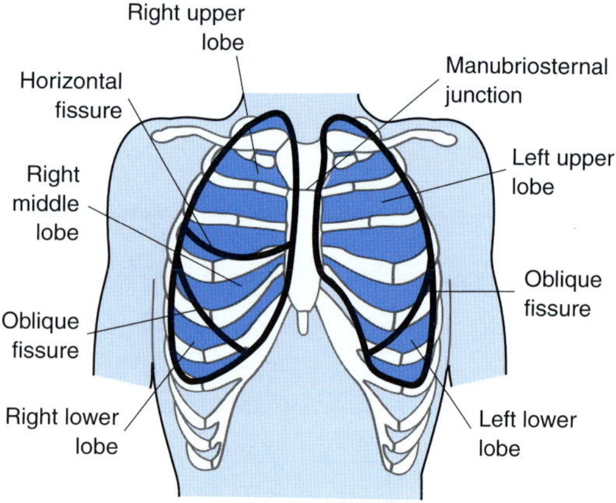

Figure 3.1 Lung markings – anterior view.

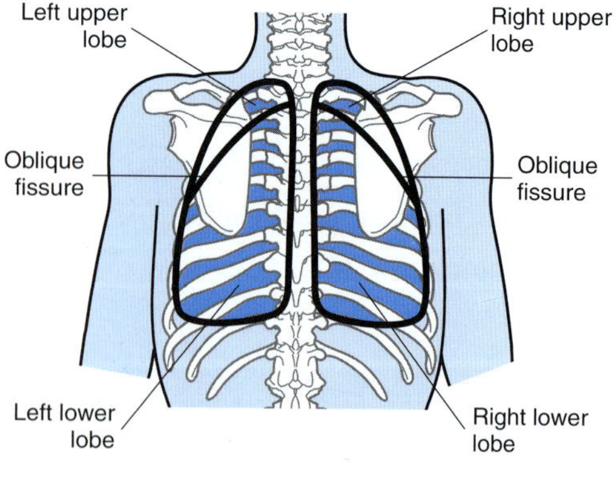

Figure 3.2 Lung markings – posterior view.

Useful lung markings*

Apex	Anterior – 2.5 cm above clavicles Posterior – T1
Lower borders	Anterior – sixth rib Posterior – T10/11 Mid-axilla – eighth rib
Tracheal bifurcation	Anterior – manubriosternal junction Posterior – T4
Right horizontal fissure	Anterior – fourth rib (above the nipple)
Oblique fissures	Anterior – sixth rib (below the nipple) Posterior – T2/3
Left diaphragm	Anterior – sixth rib Posterior – T10 Mid-axilla – eighth rib
Right diaphragm	Anterior – fifth rib Posterior – T9 Mid-axilla – eighth rib

*These lung markings are approximate and can vary between individuals.

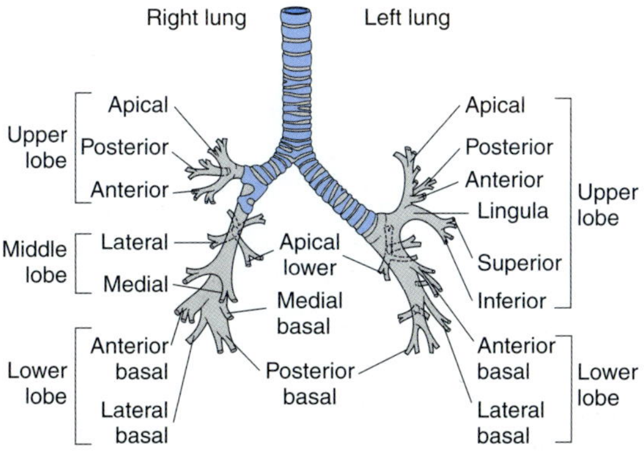

Figure 3.3 Anterior view of bronchial tree.

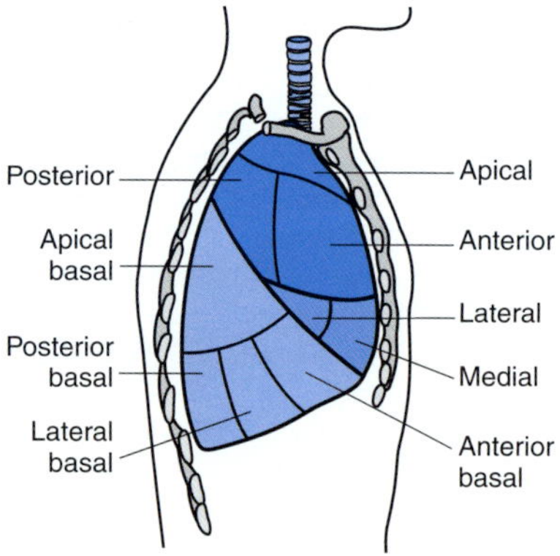

Figure 3.4 Bronchopulmonary segments – right lateral view.

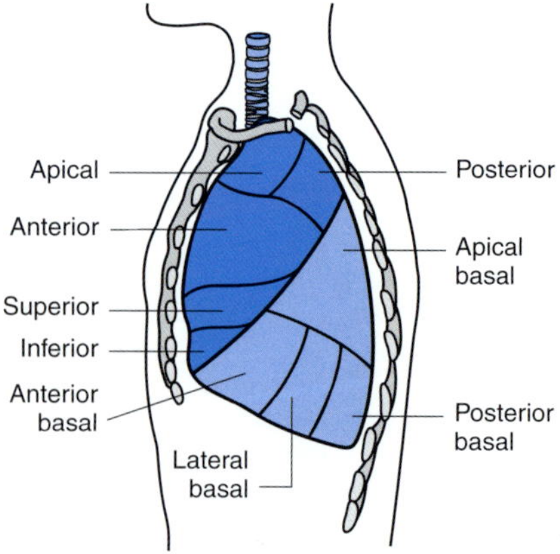

Figure 3.5 Bronchopulmonary segments – left lateral view.

Respiratory volumes and capacities

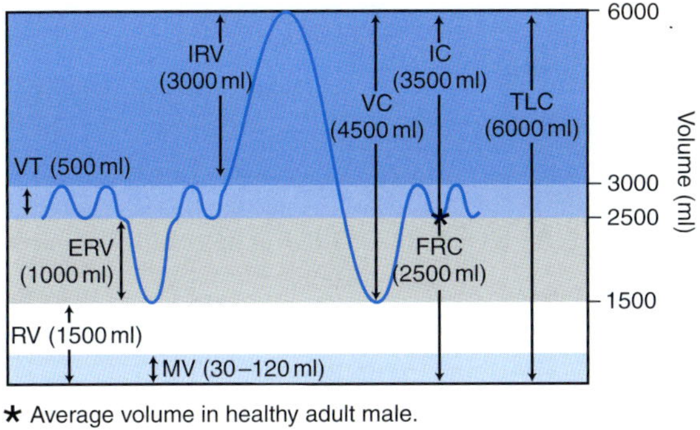

Figure 3.6 Respiratory volumes and capacities.

Lung volumes

VT (tidal volume)

Volume of air inhaled or exhaled during a single normal breath

Value: 500 ml

IRV (inspiratory reserve volume)

Maximum amount of air that can be inspired on top of a normal tidal inspiration

Value: 3000 ml

ERV (expiratory reserve volume)

Maximum amount of air that can be exhaled following a normal tidal expiration

Value: 1000 ml

RV (residual volume)

Volume of air remaining in the lungs after a maximal expiration
Value: 1500 ml

MV (minimal volume)

The amount of air that would remain if the lungs collapsed
Value: 30–120 ml

Lung capacities

A capacity is the combination of two or more lung volumes

TLC (total lung capacity)

Total volume of your lungs at the end of maximal inspiration

$TLC = VT + IRV + ERV + RV$

Value: 6000 ml

VC (vital capacity)

Maximum amount of air that can be inspired and expired in a single breath

$VC = VT + IRV + ERV$

Value: 4500 ml

IC (inspiratory capacity)

The maximum volume of air that can be inspired after a normal tidal expiration

$IC = VT + IRV$

Value: 3500 ml

FRC (functional residual capacity)

Volume of air remaining in the lungs at the end of a normal tidal expiration

$FRC = ERV + RV$

Value: 2500 ml

Chest X-rays

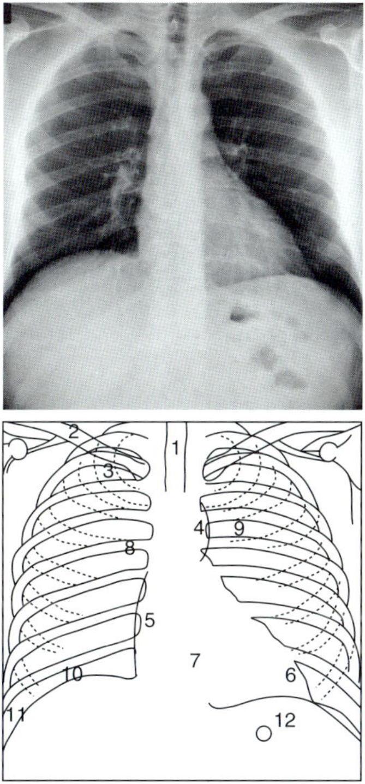

1 Air in the trachea	7 Right ventricle
2 Clavicle	8 Right hilum
3 1st rib	9 Left hilum
4 Aortic arch	10 Right hemidiaphragm
5 Right atrium	11 Costophrenic angle
6 Left ventricle	12 Gastric bubble

Figure 3.7 (a) Normal PA chest X-ray (Pryor & Prasad); (b) structures normally visible on X-ray.

Analysing chest X-rays

Adopt a systematic approach when analysing X-rays. You should check the following:

Patient's details

- Name, date and time of X-ray

Is it anteroposterior (AP) or posteroanterior (PA)? Supine or erect?

- AP X-rays are taken using a mobile machine with the patient in supine. The heart appears larger and the scapulae are visible
- PA X-rays are taken in the radiology department with the patient standing erect. The quality is generally better and the scapulae are out of the way

Is the patient positioned symmetrically?

- The medial ends of the clavicle should be equidistant from the adjacent vertebral body. If the patient is rotated the position of the heart, spine and rib cage may appear distorted

Degree of inspiration

- On full inspiration the sixth or seventh rib should intersect the midpoint of the right hemidiaphragm anteriorly or the ninth rib posteriorly

Exposure

- If the film appears too dark it is overpenetrated (overexposed)
- If the film appears too light it is underpenetrated (underexposed)
  Think of toast: dark is overdone and white is underdone
- The spinous processes of the cervical and upper thoracic vertebra should be visible, as should the outline of the mid-thoracic vertebral bodies

Extrathoracic soft tissues

- Surgical emphysema is often seen in the supraclavicular areas, around the armpit and the lateral chest wall
- The lateral wall of the chest may be obscured by breast shadows

Invasive medical equipment

- Note the position and presence of any tubes, cannulas, electrodes, etc.
- The tip of the endotracheal tube should lie about 2 cm above the carina

Bony structures

- Check for fractures, deformities and osteoporosis

Intercostal spaces

- Small intercostal spaces and steeply sloping ribs indicate reduced lung volume
- Large intercostal spaces and horizontal ribs indicate hyperinflation

Trachea

- Lies centrally with the lower third inclining slightly to the right
- Deviation of the trachea indicates mediastinal shift. It shifts towards collapse and away from tumours, pleural effusions and pneumothoracies
- Bifurcation into the left and right bronchi is normally seen. The right bronchus follows the line of the trachea whereas the left bronchus branches off at a more acute angle

Hila

- Made up of the pulmonary vessels and lymph nodes
- The left and right hilum should be roughly equal in size, though the left hilum appears slightly higher than the right. Their silhouette should be sharp

Heart

- On a PA film the diameter of the heart is usually less than half the total diameter of the thorax. In the majority of cases, one-third of the cardiac shadow lies on the right and two-thirds on the left, which should be sharply defined. The density of both sides should be equal. The heart may appear bigger on an AP film or if the patient is rotated

Diaphragm

- The right side of the diaphragm is about 2 cm higher than the left because the right lobe of the liver is situated directly underneath it. Both hemidiaphragms should be dome shaped and sharply defined
- The costophrenic angle is where the diaphragm meets the ribs
- The cardiophrenic angle is where the diaphragm meets the heart

Auscultation

Auscultation should be conducted in a systematic manner, comparing the same area on the left and right side while visualizing the underlying lung structures. Ideally patients should be sitting upright and be asked to breathe through the mouth to reduce nose turbulence.

Breath sounds

Normal

More prominent at the top of the lungs and centrally, with the volume decreasing towards the bases and periphery. Expiration is shorter and quieter than inspiration and follows inspiration without a pause.

Abnormal (bronchial breathing)

Similar to the breath sounds heard when listening over the trachea. They are typically loud and harsh and can be heard throughout inspiration and expiration. Expiration is longer than inspiration and there is a pause between the two. They occur if air is replaced by solid tissue, which transmits sound more clearly. Caused by consolidation, areas of collapse, pleural effusion, tumour.

Diminished

Breath sounds will be reduced if air entry is compromised by either an obstruction or a decrease in airflow. Caused by pneumothorax, pleural effusion, emphysema, collapse with occluded bronchus, inability to breathe deeply, obesity.

Added sounds

Crackles

Heard when airways that have been narrowed or closed, usually by secretions, are suddenly forced open on inspiration. Usually classified as fine (originating from distal airways) or coarse (from proximal airways). They can be further defined as being early, middle or late, depending on when they are heard on inspiration.

Wheeze

Caused by air being forced through narrowed airways. Described as either high or low pitched and monophonic (single note) or polyphonic (where several airways may be obstructed). Airway narrowing can be caused by bronchospasm, mucosal oedema or sputum retention. An expiratory wheeze with prolonged expiration is usually indicative of bronchospasm, while a low-pitched wheeze throughout inspiration and expiration is normally caused by secretions.

Pleural rub

If the pleural surfaces are inflamed or infected they become rough and rub together creating a creaking or grating sound.

Voice sounds

In normal lung tissue, voice sounds are indistinct and unintelligible. When there is consolidation, sound is transmitted more clearly and loudly and speech can be distinguished. Voice sounds can be heard through a stethoscope (vocal resonance) or felt by hand (vocal fremitus). To test voice sounds patients can be asked to say '99' repeatedly.

Percussion note

Elicited by placing the middle finger of one hand firmly in the space between the ribs and tapping it sharply with the middle finger of the other hand.

The pitch of the note is determined by whether the lungs contain air, solid or fluid and will either sound normal, resonant, dull or stony dull.

Resonant = hyperinflated chest or pneumothorax
Dull = consolidated lung or areas of collapse
Stony dull = pleural effusion

Interpreting blood gas values

Arterial blood analysis	Reference ranges
pH	7.35–7.45 pH
PaO_2	10.7–13.3 kPa (80–100 mmHg)
$PaCO_2$	4.7–6.0 kPa (35–45 mmHg)
HCO_3^-	22–26 mmol/L
Base excess	−2 to +2

Assessing acid–base disorders

Assessing acid–base disorders involves examining the pH, $PaCO_2$ and HCO_3^-:

- pH – a low pH (<7.4) indicates a tendency towards acidosis, a high pH (>7.4) indicates a tendency towards alkalosis
- $PaCO_2$ – an increase in $PaCO_2$ leads to acidosis, a decrease to alkalosis
- HCO_3^- – an increase in HCO_3^- leads to alkalosis, a decrease to acidosis

Assessment

1. Establish whether the patient's pH is acidotic, alkalotic or normal
2. If the pH is acidotic establish whether this is due to:
   - increased $PaCO_2$ – indicating respiratory acidosis
   - decreased HCO_3^- – indicating metabolic acidosis
3. If the pH is alkalotic establish whether this is due to:
   - decreased $PaCO_2$ – indicating respiratory alkalosis
   - increased HCO_3^- – indicating metabolic acidosis
4. If the pH is within normal range the original abnormality can be identified by comparing the pH to the $PaCO_2$ and the HCO_3^-. If the pH is below 7.4 (tending towards acid) then the component that correlates with acidosis (increased $PaCO_2$ or decreased HCO_3^-) is the cause and the other is the compensation. Likewise if the pH is above 7.4 (tending towards alkaline) the component that correlates with alkalosis (decreased $PaCO_2$ or increased HCO_3^-) is the cause and the other is the compensation.

Simple acid–base disorders

	pH	$PaCO_2$	HCO_3^-
Respiratory acidosis			
Uncompensated	↓	↑	N
Compensated	N	↑	↑

	pH	$PaCO_2$	HCO_3^-
Respiratory alkalosis Uncompensated Compensated	 ↑ N	 ↓ ↓	 N ↓
Metabolic acidosis Uncompensated Compensated	 ↓ N	 N ↓	 ↓ ↓
Metabolic alkalosis Uncompensated Compensated	 ↑ N	 N ↑	 ↑ ↑

↓ = decreased; ↑ = increased; N = normal

Base excess

Allows assessment of the metabolic component of acid–base disturbances and therefore the degree of renal compensation that has occurred. A base deficit (less than −2) indicates a metabolic acidosis and a base excess (greater than +2) correlates with metabolic alkalosis.

Respiratory failure

Broadly defined as an inability of the respiratory system to maintain blood gas values within normal ranges. There are two types:

Type I (hypoxaemic respiratory failure)

A decreased PaO_2 (hypoxaemia) with a normal or low $PaCO_2$ due to inadequate gas exchange. Causes include pneumonia, emphysema, fibrosing alveolitis, severe asthma and adult respiratory distress syndrome.

Defined as $PaO_2 < 8$ kPa (60 mmHg)

Type II (ventilatory failure)

A decreased PaO_2 with an increased $PaCO_2$ (hypercapnia) caused by hypoventilation. Causes include neuromuscular disorders (e.g. muscular dystrophy, Guillain–Barré), lung diseases (e.g. asthma, COPD), drug-related respiratory drive depression and injuries to the chest wall.

Defined as $PaO_2 < 8$ kPa (60 mmHg), $PaCO_2 > 6.7$ kPa (50 mmHg)

Arterial blood gas classification of respiratory failure

	pH	$PaCO_2$	HCO_3^-
Acute	↓	↑	N
Chronic	N	↑	↑
Acute on chronic	↓	↑	↑

↓ = decreased; ↑ = increased; N = normal

Nasal cannula

To convert litres of O_2 to FiO_2
RA ≈ 21% FiO_2
1 Lpm ≈ 24% FiO_2
2 Lpm ≈ 28% FiO_2
3 Lpm ≈ 32% FiO_2
4 Lpm ≈ 36% FiO_2
5 Lpm ≈ 40% FiO_2
6 Lpm ≈ 44% FiO_2

RA = room air

>6 Lpm has little effect on FiO_2 and may lead to irritation and drying of the nasal mucosa

These are approximate figures as the patient's flow rates, ability to breathe through the nose, and build up of nasal mucus may all affect the amount of oxygen received. As a general rule the FiO_2 is raised by 3–4% for each litre of oxygen.

Sputum analysis (Middleton & Middleton 2002, with permission)

	Description	**Causes**
Saliva	Clear watery fluid	
Mucoid	Opalescent or white	Chronic bronchitis without infection, asthma
Muco-purulent	Slightly discoloured, but frank pus	Bronchiectasis, cystic fibrosis, pneumonia
Purulent	Thick, viscous: – yellow – dark green/brown – rusty – redcurrant jelly	 *Haemophilus* *Pseudomonas* *Pneumococcus, mycoplasma* *Klebsiella*
Frothy	Pink or white	Pulmonary oedema
Haemoptysis	Ranging from blood specks to frank blood, old blood (dark brown)	Infection (tuberculosis, bronchiectasis), infarction, carcinoma, vasculitic, trauma, also coagulation disorders, cardiac disease
Black	Black specks in mucoid secretions	Smoke inhalation (fires, tobacco, heroin), coal dust

Modes of mechanical ventilation

Controlled mechanical ventilation (CMV)

Delivers a preset number of breaths to the patient at a preset tidal volume, pressure and flow rate. The ventilator performs all the work of breathing – the patient cannot trigger the machine or breathe spontaneously. Patients on CMV are sedated and paralysed.

Assist/control ventilation (ACV)

Spontaneously breathing patients trigger a breath and the ventilator delivers gas at a preset tidal volume or preset pressure. The ventilator will initiate a breath automatically should the patient fail to trigger within a preset time.

Intermittent mandatory ventilation (IMV)

Delivers a preset number of breaths at a preset tidal volume and flow rate but allows the patient to take spontaneous breaths between machine-delivered breaths.

Synchronized intermittent mandatory ventilation (SIMV)

Synchronizes breaths from the ventilator with the patient's spontaneous breaths. If the patient fails to take a spontaneous breath within a set time the ventilator delivers a mandatory breath at either a preset tidal volume (SIMV/volume cycled) or preset inspiratory pressure (SIMV/pressure cycled).

Pressure support (PS)

Patients breathe spontaneously triggering the ventilator to deliver a set level of positive pressure to assist air entry and reduce the work of breathing. The patient controls the tidal volume, respiratory rate and flow rate. Pressure support can be added to SIMV to compensate for the resistance from the endotracheal tube making it easier for the patient to breathe.

High-frequency ventilation

This mode of ventilation does not try to imitate normal physiological breathing. Instead it delivers low tidal volumes at high respiratory rates. This results in lower airway pressures, thereby reducing the risk of complications associated with barotrauma. There are three types:

- *High-frequency positive pressure ventilation*: delivers small tidal volumes at high respiratory rates (60–100 breaths/min)
- *High-frequency oscillation ventilation*: oscillates small bursts of gas to and fro at high rates (up to 3000 cycles/min)
- *High-frequency jet ventilation*: delivers a short, rapid, high-pressure jet to the airways through a small-bore cannula (100–600 cycles/min).

Continuous positive airway pressure (CPAP)

A high flow of gas delivered continuously throughout inspiration and expiration during spontaneous breathing. The alveoli and smaller airways are splinted open, increasing lung volume at the end of expiration (i.e. the functional residual capacity), thereby reversing atelectasis and improving gas exchange. It also increases lung compliance and decreases the work of breathing.

Bilevel positive airway pressure (BiPAP)

Similar to CPAP, positive airway pressure is delivered throughout inspiration and expiration during spontaneous breathing but the level of positive airway pressure alters between inspiration and expiration. A higher level is delivered during inspiration and a lower level during expiration. The alteration between pressure levels is synchronized with the patient's breathing.

This is usually by means of a trigger that is sensitive to changes in flow (triggered or spontaneous mode) but the ventilator can also deliver breaths should the patient fail to inhale spontaneously (timed/spontaneous mode or assist-control mode).

Non-invasive ventilation (NIV)

NIV is the provision of ventilatory support without intubation, usually via a mask or similar device, to the upper airway. Positive pressure ventilation is the most common form though negative pressure ventilation is used in some situations. Positive pressure devices may be pressure, volume or time controlled and the following modes may be used: controlled mechanical ventilation, assist/control ventilation, pressure support ventilation (assisted spontaneous breathing), CPAP, BiPAP and proportional assist ventilation.

Contraindications to NIV (British Thoracic Society 2002, with permission)

- Facial trauma/burns
- Recent facial, upper airway or upper gastrointestinal tract surgery*
- Fixed obstruction of the upper airway
- Inability to protect airway*
- Life-threatening hypoxaemia*
- Haemodynamic instability*
- Severe co-morbidity*
- Impaired consciousness*
- Confusion/agitation*
- Vomiting
- Bowel obstruction*
- Copious respiratory secretions*
- Focal consolidation on chest radiograph*
- Undrained pneumothorax*

* NIV may be used, despite the presence of these contraindications, if it is to be the 'ceiling' of treatment.

Cardiorespiratory monitoring

Arterial blood pressure (ABP)

Measured via an intra-arterial cannula which allows continuous monitoring of the patient's blood pressure and also provides an access for arterial blood sampling and blood gas analysis.

Normal value: 95/60–140/90 mmHg in adults (increases gradually with age)

Hypertension: >145/95 mmHg

Hypotension: <90/60 mmHg

Cardiac output (CO)

Amount of blood pumped into the aorta each minute.

$CO = HR \times SV$

Normal value: 4–8 L/min

Cardiac index (CI)

Cardiac output related to body size. Body surface area is calculated by using the patient's weight and height and a nomogram. Allows reliable comparison between patients of different sizes.

$CI = CO \div \text{body surface area}$

Normal value: 2.5–4 $L/min/m^2$

Central venous pressure (CVP)

Measured via a central venous cannula inserted into the internal or external jugular vein or subclavian vein with the tip resting close to the right atrium within the superior vena cava. Provides information on circulating blood volume, the effectiveness of the heart to pump that volume, vascular tone and venous return.

Normal value: 3–15 cmH_2O

Cerebral perfusion pressure (CPP)

Pressure required to ensure adequate blood supply to the brain.

CPP = MAP − ICP

Normal value: >70 mmHg

Ejection fraction (EF)

The stroke volume (SV) as a percentage of the total volume of the ventricle prior to systolic contraction, i.e. end diastolic volume (EDV).

EF = SV ÷ EDV

Normal value: 65–75%

Heart rate (HR)

The number of times the heart contracts in a minute.
Normal value: 50–100 bpm
Tachycardia: >100 bpm at rest
Bradycardia: <50 bpm at rest

Intracranial pressure (ICP)

Pressure exerted by the brain tissue, cerebrospinal fluid and blood volume within the rigid skull and meninges. Neurological insults such as space-occupying lesions, cerebral oedema, hydrocephalus, cerebral haemorrhage, hypoxia and infection cause this pressure to rise resulting in a decreased blood supply to the brain. When treating patients with raised ICP minimize handling and ensure that the head is maintained in midline and raised 15–30° from supine. A marked degree of hip flexion should be avoided to ensure optimal circulation and prevent potential increase in ICP.
Normal value: 0–10 mmHg

Mean arterial pressure (MAP)

Measures the average pressure of blood being pushed through the circulatory system. It relates to cardiac output and systemic vascular resistance and reflects tissue perfusion pressure.

$MAP = (diastolic\ BP \times 2) + (systolic\ BP) \div 3$

Normal value: 80–100 mmHg
<60 mmHg indicates inadequate circulation to the vital organs

Oxygen saturation (SpO_2)

Arterial oxygen saturation is measured using non-invasive pulse oximetry.
Normal value: 95–98%

Pulmonary artery pressure (PAP)

A pulmonary artery balloon catheter (Swan–Ganz) is inserted via the CVP catheter route and floated into the pulmonary artery via the right ventricle. The PAP measures pressures of the blood in the vena cava, right atrium and right ventricle and provides a measure of the ability of the right side of the heart to push blood through the lungs and to the left side of the heart.
Normal value: 15–25/8–15 mmHg
Mean value: 10–20 mmHg

Pulmonary artery wedge pressure (PAWP)

Similar to PAP but the Swan–Ganz catheter is moved further along until it wedges in a small pulmonary artery. The balloon tip is inflated to occlude the artery in order to allow measurement of the pressure in the pulmonary capillaries in front of it and the left atrium. PAWP is also known as pulmonary capillary wedge pressure (PCWP).
Normal value: 6–12 mmHg

Respiratory rate (RR)

Number of breaths taken in a minute.
Normal value: 12–16 breaths/min
Tachypnoea: >20 breaths/min
Bradypnoea: <10 breaths/min

Stroke volume (SV)

The amount of blood ejected from the ventricles during each systolic contraction. Affected by preload (amount of tension on the ventricular wall before it contracts), afterload (resistance that the ventricle must work against when it contracts) and contractility (force of contraction generated by the myocardium).

$SV = (CO \times 1000) \div HR$

Normal value: 60–130 ml/beat

Systemic vascular resistance (SVR)

Evaluates the vascular component of afterload in the left ventricle. Vasocontriction will increase systemic vascular resistance while vasodilation will decrease it.

$SVR = (MAP - CVP \div CO) \times 79.9$

Normal value: 800–1400 dyne/sec/cm^{-5}

Biochemical and haematological studies

Blood serum studies

Test	Function	Interpretation
Sodium 136–145 mmol/L	Regulates body's water balance, maintains acid–base balance and electrical nerve potentials	*Increased (hypernatraemia)*: excessive fluid loss or salt intake, water deprivation, diabetes insipidus, excess aldosterone secretion, diarrhoea *Decreased (hyponatraemia)*: kidney disease, excessive water intake, adrenal insufficiency, diarrhoea, profuse sweating, diuretics, congestive heart failure, inappropriate secretion of ADH
Potassium 3.6–5.0 mmol/L	Nerve impulse transmission, contractility of myocardial, skeletal and smooth muscle	*Increased (hyperkalaemia)*: renal failure, increased intake of potassium, metabolic acidosis, tissue trauma (e.g. burns and infection), potassium-sparing diuretics, adrenal insufficiency *Decreased (hypokalaemia)*: potassium-wasting diuretics, vomiting, diarrhoea, metabolic alkalosis, excess aldosterone secretion, polyuria, profuse sweating

Calcium 2.1–2.6 mmol/L	Nerve impulse transmission, bone and teeth formation, skeletal and myocardial muscle contraction, activation of enzymes, blood coagulation, cell division and repair, membrane structure and absorption of vitamin B_{12}	*Increased (hypercalcaemia)*: hyperparathyroidism, malignancy, Paget's disease, osteoporosis, immobilization, renal failure *Decreased (hypocalcaemia)*: hypoparathyroidism, vitamin D deficiency, acute pancreatitis, low blood albumin, low blood magnesium, large transfusion of citrated blood, increased urine excretion, respiratory acidosis
Magnesium 0.7–1.0 mmol/L	Neuromuscular transmission, cofactor in activation of many enzyme systems for cellular metabolism (e.g. phosphorylation of glucose, production and functioning of ATP), regulation of protein synthesis	*Increased (hypermagnesaemia)*: renal failure, adrenal insufficiency, excessive oral or parenteral intake of magnesium, severe hydration *Decreased (hypomagnesaemia)*: excessive loss from GIT (diarrhoea, nasogastric suction, pancreatitis), decreased gut absorption, renal disease, long-term use of certain drugs (e.g. diuretics, digoxin), chronic alcoholism, increased aldosterone secretion, polyuria
Phosphate 0.8–1.4 mmol/L	Bone formation, formation of high energy compounds (e.g. ATP), nucleic acid synthesis, enzyme activation	*Increased (hyperphosphataemia)*: renal failure, hypoparathyroidism, chemotherapy, excessive phosphorus intake

Test	Function	Interpretation
		Decreased (hypophosphataemia): Hyperparathyroidism, chronic alcoholism, diabetes, respiratory alkalosis, excessive glucose ingestion, hypoalimentation, chronic use of antacids
Creatinine 55–150 µmol/L	End-product of normal muscle metabolism	*Increased*: renal failure, urinary obstruction, muscle disease *Decreased*: pregnancy, muscle wasting
Urea 2.5–6.5 mmol/L	Waste product of metabolism	*Increased*: renal failure, decreased renal perfusion because of heart disease, shock *Decreased*: high carbohydrate/low protein diets, late pregnancy, malabsorption, severe liver damage
Glucose 3.6–5.8 mmol/L	Metabolized in the cells to produce energy	*Increased*: diabetes mellitus, Cushing's disease, patients on steroid therapy *Decreased*: severe liver disease, adrenocortical insufficiency, drug toxicity, digestive diseases
Albumin 36–47 g/L	Most abundant plasma protein. Maintains osmotic pressure of the blood. Transports blood constituents such as fatty acids, hormones, enzymes, drugs and other substances	*Increased*: relative increase with haemoconcentration, where there is severe loss of body water *Decreased*: malnutrition, malabsorption, severe liver disease, renal disease, GI conditions causing excessive loss, thyrotoxicosis, chemotherapy, Cushing's disease

Lactate dehydrogenase 230–460 U/L	Enzyme that converts pyruvic acid into lactate. High levels found in myocardial and skeletal muscle, the liver, lungs, kidneys and red blood cells	*Increased*: tissue damage due to myocardial infarction, liver disease, renal disease, cellular damage in trauma, hypothyroidism, muscular diseases
Creatine kinase *Men* 30–200 U/L *Women* 30–150 U/L	Enzyme found in heart, brain and skeletal muscle. Increased when one of these areas is stressed or damaged. Testing for a specific creatine kinase isoenzyme indicates area of damage (e.g. raised CK-MB indicates damage to heart)	*Increased*: heart (myocardial infarction, myocarditis, open heart surgery), brain (brain cancer, trauma, seizure) and skeletal muscle damage (intramuscular injections, trauma, surgery, strenuous exercise, muscular dystrophy)
C-reactive protein <7 mg/L	Protein produced in the acute inflammatory phase of injury. Index for monitoring disease activity	*Increased*: pyrexia, all inflammatory conditions (e.g. rheumatoid arthritis, pneumococcal pneumonia), trauma, during late pregnancy
Bilirubin 2–17 μmol/L	Pigment produced by the breakdown of haem	*Increased*: hepatitis, biliary tract obstruction, haemolysis, haematoma *Decreased*: iron deficiency, anaemia

Haematological studies (data from Matassarin-Jacobs 1997, with permission of W B Saunders; Wilkins et al 2000, with permission of Mosby)

Test	Assesses	Interpretation
Red blood cell count (RBC) *Men* 4.5–6.5 $\times 10^{12}$/L *Women* 3.8–5.3 $\times 10^{12}$/L	Blood loss, anaemia, polycythaemia (increase in Hb concentration of the blood)	*Increased*: polycythaemia vera, dehydration, cardiac and pulmonary disorders characterized by cyanosis, acute poisoning *Decreased*: leukaemia, anaemia, fluid overload, haemorrhage
White blood cell count (WBC) 4.0–11.0 $\times 10^{9}$/L	Detects infection or inflammation. Monitors response to radiation and chemotherapy	*Increased*: leukaemia, tissue necrosis, infection *Decreased*: bone marrow suppression
White blood cell differential *Neutrophils* 1.5–7.0 $\times 10^{9}$/L *Lymphocytes* 1.2–3.5 $\times 10^{9}$/L *Monocytes* 0.2–1.0 $\times 10^{9}$/L	Evaluates body's ability to resist infection. Detects and classifies leukaemia	*Increased* (Wilkins et al 2000): Neutrophil – bacterial infection, inflammation Eosinophil – allergic reaction, parasitic infection Lymphocyte – viral infection Monocyte – chronic infections, malignancies Basophil – myeloproliferative disorders

Eosinophils $0.0–0.4 \times 10^9$/L *Basophils* $0.0–0.2 \times 10^9$/L		
Packed cell volume (PCV)/ haematocrit (Hct) *Men* 0.40–0.54 l/L *Women* 0.35–0.47 l/L	Blood loss and fluid balance	*Increased*: polycythaemia, dehydration *Decreased*: anaemia, acute blood loss, haemodilution
Haemoglobin (Hb) *Men* 130–180 g/L *Women* 115–165 g/L	Anaemia and polycythaemia	*Increased*: polycythaemia, dehydration *Decreased*: anaemia, recent haemorrhage, fluid overload
Platelets (Plt) $150–400 \times 10^9$/L	Severity of thrombocytopenia	*Increased*: polycythaemia vera, splenectomy, malignancy *Decreased*: anaemias, infiltrative bone marrow disease, haemolytic disorders, disseminated intravascular coagulopathy, idiopathic thrombocytopenic purpura, viral infections, AIDS, splenomegaly, with radiation or chemotherapy

Coagulation studies

Test	Description	Interpretation
Prothrombin time (PT) 12–16 sec	Measures extrinsic clotting time of blood plasma and clotting factor deficiencies	*Increased*: bile duct obstruction, liver disease, disseminated intravascular coagulation, malabsorption of nutrients from GI tract, vitamin K deficiency, warfarin therapy, factor I (fibrinogen), II (prothrombin), V, VII, X deficiency
Activated partial thromboplastin time (APTT) 30–40 sec	Measures intrinsic clotting time of blood plasma and clotting factor deficiencies	*Increased*: liver disease, disseminated intravascular coagulation, factor XI, VIII (haemophilia A) and IX (haemophilia B) deficiency, hypofibrinogenaemia, malabsorption from GI tract, heparin or warfarin therapy
International normalized ratio (INR) 0.89–1.10	Standardized measure of clotting time derived from the PT. An INR of 1 is assigned to the time it takes for normal blood to clot	*Increased*: indicates excessive bleeding tendencies *Decreased*: indicates increased risk of thrombosis

Values vary from laboratory to laboratory, depending on testing methods used. These reference ranges should be used as a guide only. All reference ranges apply to adults only; they may differ in children.

Respiratory pathologies

Acute respiratory distress syndrome (ARDS)

ARDS can be caused by a wide variety of factors including pneumonia, sepsis, smoke inhalation, aspiration, major trauma and burns. As a result, the body launches an inflammatory response that affects the alveolar epithelium and pulmonary capillaries. In ARDS the alveolar walls break down and the pulmonary capillaries become more permeable allowing plasma and blood to leak into the interstitial and alveolar spaces, while at the same time the capillaries become blocked with cellular debris and fibrin. The lungs become heavy, stiff and waterlogged and the alveoli collapse. This leads to ventilation/perfusion mismatch and hypoxaemia and patients normally require mechanical ventilatory support to achieve adequate gas exchange. Symptoms usually develop within 24–48 hours after the original injury or illness but can develop 5–10 days later.

Asthma

A chronic inflammatory disease of the airways that makes them hyper-responsive to a wide range of stimuli including allergens, pollution, infection, exercise and stress. As a result the airways narrow, leading to coughing, wheezing, chest tightness and difficulty breathing. These symptoms can range from mild to severe; and may even result in death.

Bronchiectasis

Dilatation and destruction of the bronchi as a result of recurrent inflammation or infection. It may be present from birth (congenital bronchiectasis) or acquired as a result of another disorder (acquired bronchiectasis). Causes of infection include impaired mucociliary clearance due to congenital disorders such as primary ciliary dyskinesia or cystic fibrosis as well as bronchial obstruction and impaired inflammatory response, either acquired after a severe episode of inflammation or secondary to immunodeficiency. The inability of the airways to clear secretions in the bronchi leads to a vicious circle of infection, damage and obstruction of the bronchi. Clinical features include: productive cough, episodic fever, pleuritic pain and night sweats. Patients may develop pneumothorax, respiratory and heart failure, emphysema and haemoptysis.

Bronchitis

An inflammation of the bronchi. Acute bronchitis is commonly associated with viral respiratory infections, i.e. the common cold or influenza, causing a productive cough, fever and wheezing. Chronic bronchitis is defined as a cough productive of sputum for 3 months per year for more than 2 consecutive years. It is characterized by inflammation of the airways leading to permanent fibrotic changes, excessive mucus production and thickening of the bronchial wall. This results in sputum retention and narrowing and obstruction of the airways. In severe cases irreversible narrowing of the airways leads to dyspnoea, cyanosis, hypoxia, hypercapnia and heart failure. These patients are often described as 'blue bloaters'.

Chronic obstructive pulmonary disease (COPD)

An umbrella term for respiratory disorders that lead to obstruction of the airways. COPD is associated mainly with emphysema and chronic bronchitis but also includes chronic asthma. Risk factors include smoking, recurrent infection, pollution and genetics. Symptoms include cough, dyspnoea, excessive mucus production and chest tightness. Patients may also develop oedema and heart failure.

Cystic fibrosis

A progressive genetic disorder of the mucus-secreting glands of the lungs, pancreas, mouth, gastrointestinal tract and sweat glands. Chloride ion secretion is reduced and sodium ion absorption is accelerated across the cell membrane resulting in the production of abnormally viscous mucus. This thickened mucus lines the intestine and lung leading to malabsorption, malnutrition and poor growth as well as recurrent respiratory infections that eventually lead to chronic lung disease. The increased concentration of sodium in sweat upsets the mineral balance in the blood and causes abnormal heart rhythms. Other complications include male infertility, diabetes mellitus, liver disease and vasculitis. The disease is eventually fatal.

Emphysema

The walls of the terminal bronchioles and alveoli are destroyed by inflammation and lose their elasticity. This causes excessive airway collapse on expiration which traps air in the enlarged alveolar sacs. This irreversible airways obstruction leads to symptoms of dyspnoea, productive cough, wheeze, recurrent respiratory infection, hyperinflated chest and weight loss. These patients are often described as 'pink puffers' who may hyperventilate, typically overusing their accessory respiratory muscles, and breathe with pursed lips in order to maintain airway pressure to decrease the amount of airway collapse.

Empyema

A collection of pus in the pleural cavity following nearby lung infection. Can cause a build-up of pressure in the lung which causes pain and shortness of breath.

Haemothorax

Blood in the pleural cavity. Commonly due to chest trauma but also found in patients with lung and pleural cancer and in those who have undergone thoracic or heart surgery.

Hyperventilation syndrome

Breathing in excess of metabolic requirements, which causes low arterial carbon dioxide levels, leading to alkalosis and changes in potassium and calcium ion distribution. As a result neuromuscular excitability and vasoconstriction occur. Clinical features include light-headedness, dizziness, chest pain, palpitations, breathlessness, tachycardia, anxiety, paraesthesia and tetanic cramps.

Interstitial lung disease

An umbrella term for a wide range of respiratory disorders characterized by inflammation and, eventually, fibrosis of the lung connective tissue. The bronchioles, alveoli and vasculature may all be affected causing the lungs to stiffen and decrease in size. Examples of interstitial lung disease include fibrosing alveolitis, asbestosis, pneumoconiosis, bird fancier's or farmer's lung, systemic lupus erythematosus, scleroderma, rheumatoid disease, cryptogenic pulmonary fibrosis and sarcoidosis.

Lung abscess

A pus-filled necrotic cavity within the lung parenchyma caused by infection.

Pleural effusion

A collection of excess fluid in the pleural cavity which can be caused by a number of mechanisms:

- increased hydrostatic pressure, e.g. congestive heart failure
- decreased plasma-oncotic pressure, e.g. cirrhosis of the liver, malnutrition
- increased capillary permeability, e.g. inflammation of the pleura
- impaired lymphatic absorption, e.g. malignancy
- communication with peritoneal space and fluid, e.g. ascites.

The fluid can either be clear/straw-coloured and have a low protein content (known as a transudate), indicating a disturbance of the normal pressure in the lung, or it can be cloudy and have a high protein content (known as an exudate), indicating infection, inflammation or malignancy.

Pleurisy

Inflammation of the pleura causing severe pain as a result of friction between their adjoining surfaces. Pain is focused at the site of the inflammation and is increased with deep inspiration and coughing. Most commonly associated with pneumonia but also tuberculosis, rheumatic diseases and chest trauma.

Pneumonia

An inflammation of the lung tissue, mostly caused by bacterial or viral infection but also by fungi or aspiration of gastric contents. Pneumonia can be divided into two types:

- Community-acquired pneumonia: most commonly caused by the bacterium *Streptococcus pneumoniae*
- Hospital-acquired pneumonia: tends to be more serious as patients are often immunocompromised and they may be infected by bacteria resistant to antibiotics.

The most common infective agents are bacteria such as *Pseudomonas*, *Klebsiella* and *Escherichia coli*. Clinical features include cough, pleuritic pain, fever, fatigue and, after a few days, purulent and/or blood-stained sputum.

Pneumothorax

A collection of air in the pleural cavity following a lesion in the lung or trauma to the chest, which causes the lung to collapse. Clinical features include acute pain, dyspnoea and decreased movement of the chest wall on the affected side. They are classified by how they are caused and divided into three types:

Spontaneous pneumothorax

Caused by rupture of an emphysematous bulla, in association with diseases such as asthma, cystic fibrosis, pneumonia or COPD. It can also develop in people with no underlying lung disease and frequently affects tall, thin young men, especially smokers.

Traumatic pneumothorax

Caused by traumatic injury to the chest, e.g. perforation of lung tissue by fractured ribs or stab wound, or during medical procedures such as insertion of central venous lines, lung biopsies or mechanical ventilation.

Tension pneumothorax

Produced when pressure within the pleural cavity increases as a result of a tear in the visceral pleura acting as a one-way valve, allowing air to enter on inspiration but preventing it from escaping on expiration. In severe cases it can cause a mediastinal shift, impairing venous return, leading to respiratory and cardiac arrest. Clinical features include increased respiratory distress, cyanosis, hypotension, tachycardia and tracheal deviation.

Primary ciliary dyskinesia

A genetic condition affecting the cilia causing abnormal ciliary activity and consequently, poor mucociliary clearance. Can be associated with situs inversus (the location of internal organs on the opposite side of the body), and where the two conditions exist together this is known as Kartagener's syndrome. Sperm can also be affected as they share a similar structure to cilia, leading to infertility in males. Clinical features include recurrent ear, sinus and chest infections, which can eventually lead to bronchiectasis.

Pulmonary embolus

A blockage in the pulmonary arterial circulation most commonly caused by blood clots from the veins in the pelvis or the legs. This causes a ventilation/perfusion imbalance and leads to arterial hypoxaemia. Risk factors include prolonged bed rest or prolonged sitting (e.g. long flights), oral contraception, surgery, pregnancy, malignancy and fractures of the femur.

Pulmonary oedema

Accumulation of fluid in the lungs. Usually caused by left ventricular failure whereby a back pressure builds up in the pulmonary veins eventually causing fluid to be pushed from the veins into the alveoli. Pulmonary oedema can also be caused by myocardial infarction, damage to mitral or aortic valves, direct lung injury, severe infection, poisoning or fluid overload. Symptoms include shortness of breath, wheezing, sweating, tachycardia and coughing up white or pink-tinged frothy secretions.

Sleep apnoea

A cessation of breathing for more than 10 seconds caused by recurrent collapse of the upper airway leading to disturbed sleep. This may occur as a result of loss of muscle tone in the pharnyx as the patient relaxes during sleep (obstructive sleep apnoea) and is usually associated with obesity or enlarged tonsils or adenoids. It may also be caused by abnormal central nervous system control of breathing (central sleep apnoea) or occur as a result of a restrictive disorder of the chest wall, e.g. scoliosis or ankylosing spondylitis, where normal use of accessory respiratory muscles is inhibited during sleep. Pulmonary hypertension, respiratory and/or heart failure may develop in severe cases.

Tuberculosis

A chronic infectious disease caused by *Mycobacterium tuberculosis* that is spread via the circulatory system or the lymph nodes. Any tissue can be infected but the lungs are the most common site as the route of infection is most often by inhalation, although it can also be by ingestion. Other sites of infection include lymph nodes, bones, gastrointestinal tract, kidneys, skin and meninges. The disease is characterized by the development of granulomas in the infected tissues. The initial lesion that develops on first exposure to the disease is referred to as the primary complex. The primary lesion can be asymptomatic and heal itself with no further complications. However, the disease can be reactivated, especially following infection, inadequate immunity and malnutrition, and is known as post-primary tuberculosis. Clinical features include cough, haemoptysis, weight loss, fatigue, fever and night sweats.

Treatment techniques

Positioning

Positioning the patient optimizes cardiovascular and cardiopulmonary function and thus oxygen transport. Correct positioning of the patient can maximize lung volume, lung compliance and the ventilation/perfusion ratio. It can also reduce the work of breathing and aid secretion removal and cough. This may involve positioning adult patients in side lying with the 'good' lung (dependent) facing down and the 'bad' lung (non-dependent) facing uppermost. Always monitor the patient after positioning.

Precautions when placing 'bad' lung up (Hough 2001)
Recent pneumonectomy
Large pleural effusion
Bronchopleural fistula
Presence of a large tumour in a main stem bronchus

Note: Positioning small children and infants to maximize ventilation/perfusion – rather than for postural drainage and removal of secretions – requires a different approach to adults. In children with unilateral lung disease the good lung should be positioned uppermost to improve oxygenation.

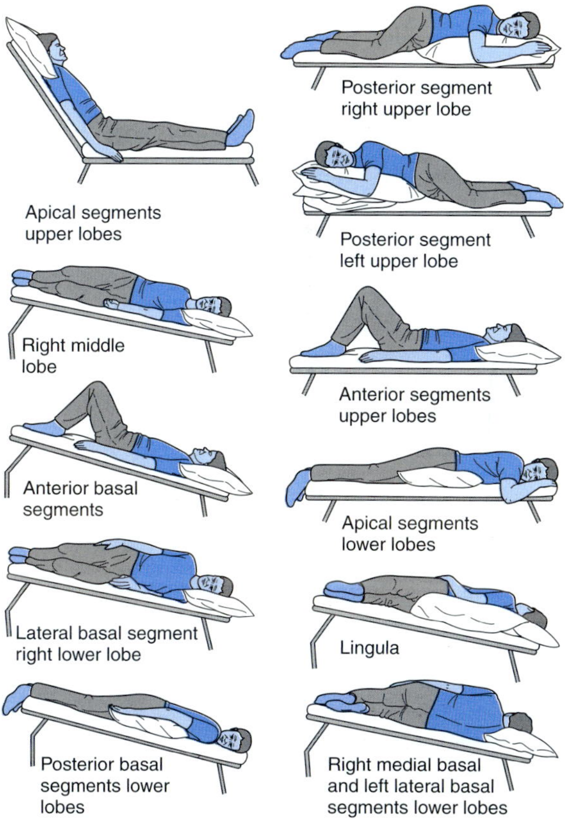

Figure 3.8 Postural drainage positions.

Postural drainage

Positioning the patient according to the anatomy of the bronchial tree in order to use gravity to assist drainage of secretions (see Fig. 3.8).

Precautions for head-down tilted positions

- Cerebral oedema/raised ICP
- Hypertension
- Cardiac failure
- Aortic and cerebral aneurysms
- Abdominal distension
- Pregnancy
- Obesity
- Gastro-oesophageal reflux
- Postoperative head and neck surgery
- Facial and neck trauma or burns
- Severe haemoptysis
- Subcutaneous/surgical emphysema

Manual chest clearance techniques

These can be used while the patient is in a postural drainage position to aid the clearance of secretions. Manual techniques include percussion, vibrations and shaking.

Precautions

- Osteoporosis
- Severe haemoptysis
- Metastatic carcinoma of the thorax
- Severe clotting disorder
- Unstable angina or cardiac arrhythmias
- Rib fractures
- Surgical emphysema
- Burns
- Pain

Active cycle of breathing technique (ACBT)
(Pryor & Webber 2002, with permission)

This consists of three different breathing techniques, namely breathing control (normal tidal breaths), thoracic expansion exercises (deep inspiratory breaths) and forced expiration technique (one or two huffs from low to high lung volume) that are repeated in cycles in order to mobilize and clear bronchial secretions. These can be used in different combinations according to the patient's needs.

Contraindications

- None if technique(s) adapted to suit the patient's condition

Airway suction

The removal of bronchial secretions through a suction catheter inserted via the nose (nasopharyngeal/NP) or mouth (oropharyngeal), or via a tracheostomy or endotracheal tube using vacuum pressure (usually in the range 8.0–20 kPa/ 60–150 mmHg).

Contraindications

- CSF leak/basal skull fracture (applies to nasopharangeal approach only)
- Stridor
- Severe bronchospasm
- Pulmonary oedema

Precautions

- Clotting disorders
- Recent oesophagectomy, lung transplant or pneumonectomy

Adverse effects

- Tracheobronchial trauma
- Bronchospasm
- Atelectasis
- Pneumothorax
- Hypoxia

- Cardiac arrhythmias
- Raised ICP

Manual hyperinflation

The use of a rebreathing bag to manually inflate the lungs in order to increase lung volume, aid the removal of secretions and assess or improve lung compliance. The peak airway pressure being delivered should not exceed 40 cmH_2O.

Contraindications

- Undrained pneumothorax
- Bullae
- Surgical emphysema
- Cardiovascular instability
- Patients at risk of barotrauma, e.g. emphysema, fibrosis
- Recent pneumonectomy/lobectomy (first 10 days)
- Severe bronchospasm (if peak airway pressure $>$40 cmH_2O)
- Unexplained haemoptysis
- Acute head injury

Adverse effects

- Barotrauma
- Haemodynamic compromise – reduced or increased blood pressure
- Cardiac arrhythmia
- Reduced oxygen saturations
- Raised intracranial pressure
- Reduced respiratory drive
- Bronchospasm

Considerations when treating patients with raised ICP

Minimize suction
Minimize manual techniques
Minimize manual hyperinflation (maintain hypocapnia)
Consider sedation/inotropic support if ICP increased or unstable
Monitor CPP: should be $>$70 mmHg

Intermittent positive pressure breathing (IPPB)

Assisted breathing using positive airway pressure to deliver gas throughout inspiration until a preset pressure is reached. Inspiration is triggered when the patient inhales and expiration is passive.

Effects

- Increases tidal volume
- Reduces work of breathing
- Assists clearance of bronchial secretions
- Improves alveolar ventilation

Contraindications

IPPB should not normally be used when any of the following conditions are present. If in doubt, medical advice should be sought.

- Undrained pneumothorax
- Facial fractures
- Acute head injury
- Large bullae
- Lung abscess
- Severe haemoptysis
- Vomiting
- Tumour or obstruction in proximal airways
- Surgical emphysema
- Recent lung and oesophageal surgery

Tracheostomies

A tracheostomy is an opening in the anterior wall of the trachea to facilitate ventilation. It is sited below the level of the vocal chords.

Indications

- Provide and maintain a patent airway when the upper airways are obstructed

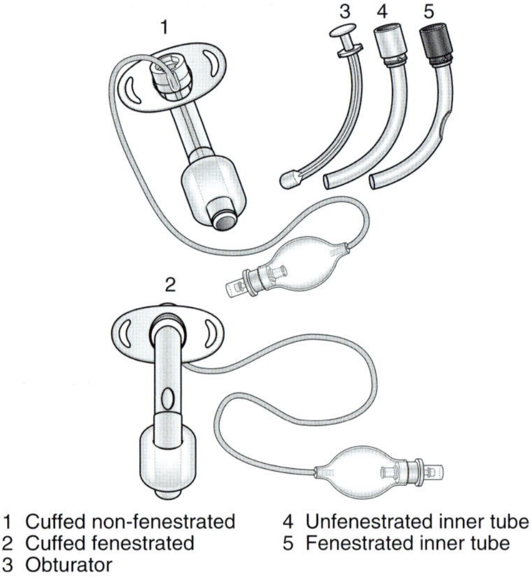

Figure 3.9 Different types of tracheostomy tubes.

- Provide access for the removal of tracheobronchial secretions
- Prevent aspiration of oral and gastric secretions in patients unable to protect their own airway
- Used in patients who need longer-term ventilation

Types of tube

Metal or plastic

- Metal tubes are used by long-term tracheostomy patients as they are more durable. They are made of either stainless steel or sterling silver and do not have connections

for respiratory equipment, e.g. a resuscitation bag. On some tubes an adaptor can be attached
- Plastic tubes are cheaper and therefore more disposable

Cuffed or uncuffed

- Cuffed tubes have an air-filled sac at their distal end. When inflated a cuffed tube provides a seal between the trachea and the tube. It protects the airway against aspiration and allows positive pressure ventilation. Patients cannot speak when the cuff is inflated, unless the tube is fenestrated
- Uncuffed tubes are used for paediatric patients as the air space around the tube can be sealed without the need for a cuff. Also used when the cuff is no longer required for ventilation, when there is no risk of aspiration, or in patients on long-term ventilation

Fenestrated

- Fenestrated tubes enable air to pass through the tube and over the vocal chords, allowing speech. They can also be used as part of the weaning process by allowing patients to breathe through the tube and use their upper airway

Single or double lumen

- Single lumen tubes consist of a single cannula. They carry the risk of becoming blocked by secretions and obstructing the airway
- Double lumen tubes consist of an inner and outer cannula. The inner cannula is removable and can be cleaned to prevent the accumulation of secretions. To allow speech the inner tube and outer tube need to be fenestrated. However, during suctioning the inner tube must be replaced with an unfenestrated tube to prevent the catheter passing through the fenestration. It must

also be in place if the patient is put on positive pressure ventilation in order to maintain pressure

Complications

- Haemorrhage
- Pneumothorax
- Tracheal tube misplacement
- End of tube blocked if pressed against carina or tracheal wall
- Surgical emphysema
- Secretions occluding tube
- Herniation of cuff causing tube blockage
- Stenosis of trachea due to granulation
- Tracheo-oesophageal fistula
- Infection of tracheostomy site
- Tracheal irritation, ulceration and necrosis caused by overinflated cuff or excessive tube movement

Respiratory assessment

Patients present with a variety of conditions and assessments need to be adapted to suit their needs. This section provides a basic framework for the subjective and objective respiratory assessment of a patient.

Database

- History of present condition
- Past medical history
- Drug history
- Family history
- Social history
  - support at home
  - home environment
  - occupation and hobbies
  - smoking

Subjective examination

- Patient's main concern
- Symptoms
  - shortness of breath
  - cough (productive or non-productive)
  - pain
  - wheeze
- Functional ability/exercise tolerance

Objective examination

Charts

- Blood pressure
- Heart rate
- Temperature
- Oxygen requirement
- Oxygen saturations
- Respiratory rate
- Weight
- Peak flow
- Fluid balance
- Urine output
- Medications

+ITU/HDU charts

- Mode of ventilation
- FiO_2
- Heart rhythm
- Pressure support/volume control
- Airway pressure
- Tidal volume
- PEEP
- CVP
- GCS
- ABGs
- Blood chemistry

Observation

- General appearance
- Position
- Oxygen therapy
- Lines and drains
- Presence of wheeze or cough
- Sputum
  - colour
  - volume
  - viscosity
- Quality of voice
- Ability to talk in full sentences
- Skin colour
- Jugular venous pressure
- Oedema
- Clubbing
- Flapping tremor
- Chest
  - shape
  - breathing pattern
  - work of breathing
  - chest wall movement
  - respiratory rate

Palpation

- Chest excursion
- Skin hydration
- Trachea
- Percussion note

Auscultation

- Breath sounds
- Added sounds
- Voice sounds

Functional ability

Exercise tolerance

References and further reading

Berne R M, Levy M N 2000 Principles of physiology, 3rd edn. Mosby, St Louis

Black J M, Matassarin-Jacobs E 1997 Medical-surgical nursing: clinical management for continuity of care, 5th edn. W B Saunders, Philadelphia

British Thoracic Society Standards of Care Committee 2002 Guidelines on non-invasive ventilation in acute respiratory failure. Thorax 57: 192–211

Bucher L, Melander S 1999 Critical care nursing. W B Saunders, Philadelphia

Frownfelter D, Dean E 1996 Principles and practice of cardiopulmonary physical therapy, 3rd edn. Mosby, St Louis

Hillegass E A, Sadowsky H S 2001 Cardiopulmonary physical therapy, 2nd edn. W B Saunders, Philadelphia

Hough A 2001 Physiotherapy in respiratory care: an evidence-based approach to respiratory and cardiac management, 3rd edn. Nelson Thornes, Cheltenham

Kozier B, Erb G, Blais K, Wilkinson J M 1998 Fundamentals of nursing: concepts, process and practice, 5th edn. Addison-Wesley Nursing, California

Martini F H 1998 Fundamentals of anatomy and physiology, 4th edn. Prentice Hall, London

Matassarin-Jacobs E 1997 Assessment of clients with haematological disorders. In: Black J M, Matassarin-Jacobs E (eds) Medical-surgical nursing: clinical management for continuity of care, 5th edn. W B Saunders, Philadelphia

Middleton S, Middleton P G 2002 Assessment and investigation of patient's problems. In: Pryor J A, Prasad S A Physiotherapy for respiratory and cardiac problems, 3rd edn. Churchill Livingstone, Edinburgh, pp. 3–25

Paz J C, West M P 2002 Acute care handbook for physical therapists, 2nd edn. Butterworth-Heinemann, Boston

Pierce L N B 1995 Guide to mechanical ventilation and intensive respiratory care. W B Saunders, Philadelphia

Potter P A, Perry A G 2003 Basic nursing: essentials for practice, 5th edn. Mosby, St Louis

Pryor J A, Prasad S A 2002 Physiotherapy for respiratory and cardiac problems, 3rd edn. Churchill Livingstone, Edinburgh

Pryor A J, Webber B A 2002 Physiotherapy techniques. In: Pryor J A, Prasad S A (eds) Physiotherapy for respiratory and cardiac problems, 3rd edn. Churchill Livingstone, Edinburgh

Smith M, Ball V 1998 Cardiovascular/respiratory physiotherapy. Mosby, London

Stillwell S B 2002 Mosby's critical care nursing reference, 3rd edn. Mosby, St Louis

Wilkins R L, Krider S J, Sheldon R L 2000 Clinical assessment in respiratory care, 4th edn. Mosby, St Louis

SECTION 3

SECTION 4

Pharmacology

Drug classes

ACE inhibitors

Angiotensin-converting enzyme (ACE) inhibitors allow blood vessels to dilate by preventing the formation of angiotensin II, a powerful artery constrictor. Used in the treatment of heart failure, hypertension, diabetic nephropathy and post-myocardial infarction.

Analgesics

Used to relieve pain and can be divided into opioids and non-opioids. Opioids block transmission of pain signals within the brain and spinal cord. They include morphine and pethidine and are used to treat moderate to severe pain arising from surgery, serious injury and terminal illness. Non-opioids are less powerful and work by blocking the production of prostaglandins, thereby preventing stimulation of nerve endings at the site of pain. Include paracetamol and non-steroidal anti-inflammatory drugs such as aspirin.

Antibiotics

Used to treat bacterial disorders ranging from minor infections to deadly diseases. Antibiotics work by destroying the bacteria or preventing them from multiplying while the body's immune system works to clear the invading organism. There are different classes of antibiotic, which include *penicillins* (amoxicillin, ampicillin, benzylpenicillin), *cephalosporins* (cefaclor, cefotaxime, cefuroxime), *macrolides* (erythromycin), *tetracyclines* (oxytetracycline, tetracycline) and *aminoglycosides* (gentamicin).

Antiepileptics

Used to prevent or terminate epileptic seizures. There are several types of epilepsy, each treated by a specific antiepileptic medication. It is therefore essential to classify the type of seizure in order to treat it effectively and minimize side-effects.

Antiemetics

Act by blocking signals to the vomiting centre in the brain which triggers the vomiting reflex. Used to prevent or treat vomiting and nausea caused by motion sickness, vertigo, digestive tract infection and to counteract the side-effects of some drugs.

β-blockers

Prevent stimulation of the β-adrenoreceptors in the heart muscle (mainly β_1-receptors) and peripheral vasculature, bronchi, pancreas and liver (mainly β_2-receptors). Used to treat hypertension, angina, myocardial infarction, arrhythmias and thyrotoxicosis. Can also be used to alleviate some symptoms of anxiety. Since blocking β-adrenoreceptors in the lungs can lead to constriction of air passages, care needs to be taken when treating patients with asthma or COPD.

Benzodiazepines

Increase the inhibitory affect of GABA, which depresses brain cell activity in the higher centres of the brain controlling consciousness. Used for anxiety, insomnia, convulsions, sedation for medical procedures and alcohol withdrawal.

Bronchodilators

Dilate the airways to assist breathing when constricted or congested with mucus. There are two main types:

Sympathomimetics (i.e. salbutamol) stimulate β_2-adrenoreceptors on the surface of bronchial smooth muscle cells causing the muscle to relax

Anticholinergics (i.e. ipratropium bromide) act by blocking the neurotransmitters that trigger muscle contraction.

Both are used to treat asthma and other conditions associated with reversible airways obstruction such as COPD.

Other drugs used as bronchodilators are *xanthines* (i.e. aminophylline) which are thought to relax bronchiole muscle and *corticosteroids* (i.e. beclometasone) which reduce airway inflammation.

Calcium channel blockers

Interfere with the transport of calcium ions through the cell walls of cardiac and vascular smooth muscle. Reduce the contractility of the heart, depress the formation and conduction of impulses in the heart and cause peripheral vasodilation. Used to treat angina, hypertension and arrhythmias.

Corticosteroids

Reduce inflammation by inhibiting the formation of inflammatory mediators, e.g. prostaglandins. Used to control many inflammatory disorders thought to be caused by excessive or inappropriate activity of the immune system, e.g. asthma, rheumatoid arthritis, lupus, eczema, as well as inflammation caused by strain and damage to muscles and tendons.

Diuretics

Work on the kidneys to increase the amount of sodium and water excreted. There are different types of diuretic that work on the nephron:

Thiazides (bendroflumethiazide/bendrofluazide)
Loop (furosemide/frusemide, bumetanide)
Potassium-sparing (amiloride, spironolactone)
Osmotic (mannitol)
Carbonic anhydrase inhibitors (acetazolamide, dorzolamide).

Used to treat hypertension (thiazides), chronic heart failure and oedema (loop diuretics, thiazides or a combination of both), glaucoma (carbonic anhydrase inhibitors or osmotic), raised intracranial pressure (osmotic).

Inotropes

Work by increasing the contractility of the heart muscle. They can be divided into three groups:

Cardiac glycosides (i.e. digoxin) assist activity of heart muscle by increasing intracellular calcium storage in myocardial cells. Used for heart failure and supraventricular arrhythmias

Sympathomimetics (i.e. dobutamine, dopamine) stimulate β_1-receptors on the heart which increase the rate and force of myocardial contraction. Provide inotropic support in infarction, cardiac surgery, cardiomyopathies, septic shock and cardiogenic shock

Phosphodiesterase inhibitors (i.e. milrinone) inactivate cyclic AMP which increases the force of myocardial contraction and relaxes vascular smooth muscle. Used to treat congestive heart failure.

Mucolytics

Reduce the viscosity of bronchopulmonary secretions by breaking down their molecular complexes. Used to treat excessive or thickened mucus secretions.

Non-steroidal anti-inflammatory drugs (NSAIDs)

Inhibit the production of prostaglandins, which are responsible for inflammation and pain following tissue damage. They are called non-steroidals to distinguish them from corticosteroids, which have a similar function. Used for inflammatory diseases, pain and pyrexia.

A–Z of drugs

Acetylcysteine (mucolytic)

Reduces the viscosity of secretions associated with impaired or abnormal mucus production. Administered with a bronchodilator as it can cause bronchospasm and inhibit ciliary function. Also used as an antidote for paracetamol overdose.
Side-effects: bronchoconstriction, nausea and vomiting.

Aciclovir (antiviral)

Used against infections caused by herpes virus (herpes simplex and varicella-zoster).
Side-effects are rare.

Adenosine (anti-arrhythmic)

Reverses supraventricular tachycardias to sinus rhythm.
Side-effects: chest pain, dyspnoea, nausea, bronchospasm, facial flush.

Adrenaline/epinephrine (sympathomimetic agent)

Used during cardiopulmonary resuscitation to stimulate heart activity and raise low blood pressure. Adrenaline (epinephrine) acts as a vasoconstrictor and is used to reduce bleeding and prolong the effects of local anaesthetic. It is also used to treat anaphylactic shock as it raises blood pressure and causes bronchodilation. Since it lowers pressure in the eye by decreasing production of aqueous humour it is used for glaucoma and eye surgery.
Side-effects: dry mouth, anxiety, restlessness, palpitations, tremor, headache, blurred vision, hypertension, tachycardias.

Alfentanil (opioid analgesic)

Fast acting, it is used as a respiratory depressant in patients needing prolonged assisted ventilation. Also used as an analgesic during surgery and to enhance anaesthesia.
Side-effects: drowsiness, nausea, vomiting, constipation, dizziness, dry mouth.

Allopurinol (anti-gout)

A prophylactic for gout and uric acid kidney stones.
Side-effects: rash, itching, nausea.

Aminophylline (xanthine)

Acts as a bronchodilator and is used for reversible airways obstruction and intravenously for acute severe asthma.
Side-effects: tachycardias, palpitations, nausea, headache, insomnia, arrhythmias, convulsions.

Amiodarone (anti-arrhythmic)

Slows nerve impulses in the heart muscle. Used to treat ventricular and supraventricular tachycardias and prevent recurrent atrial and ventricular fibrillation.
Side-effects: photosensitivity, reversible corneal depositions, liver damage and thyroid disorders.

Amitriptyline (tricyclic antidepressant)

Increases amine levels in the brain and is used to treat depressive illness and nocturnal enuresis (bedwetting) in children.
Side-effects: dry mouth, drowsiness, sweating, blurred vision, dizziness/fainting, postural hypotension, constipation.

Amoxicillin (penicillin antibiotic)

See antibiotics in Drug Classes.

Ampicillin (penicillin antibiotic)

See antibiotics in Drug Classes.

Aspirin (non-steroidal anti-inflammatory)

Used as an anti-inflammatory, as an analgesic and to reduce fever. It also inhibits thrombus formation and is used to reduce the risk of heart attacks and stroke.
Side-effects: gastric irritation leading to dyspepsia and bleeding, and wheezing in aspirin-sensitive asthmatics.

Atenolol (beta-blocker)

Used to treat hypertension, angina and arrhythmias.
Side-effects: muscle ache, fatigue, dry eyes, bradycardia and AV block, hypotension, cold peripheries.

Atracurium (non-depolarizing muscle relaxant)

Used as a muscle relaxant during surgery and to facilitate intermittent positive pressure breathing in intensive care unit.
Side-effects: skin rash, flushing, hypotension.

Atropine (antimuscarinic)

Relaxes smooth muscle and is used to treat irritable bowel syndrome. Can be used to paralyse ciliary action and enlarge the pupils during eye examinations. Also used to reverse excessive bradycardia, in cardiopulmonary resuscitation and for patients who have been poisoned with organophosphorous anticholinesterase drugs.
Side-effects: blurred vision, dry mouth, thirst, constipation, flushing, dry skin.

Azathioprine (immunosuppressant)

Prevents rejection of transplanted organs by the immune system and in a number of autoimmune and collagen diseases (including rheumatoid arthritis, polymyositis, systemic lupus).
Side-effects: nausea, vomiting, hair loss, loss of appetite, bone marrow suppression.

Beclometasone (corticosteroid)

Given by inhaler and used to control asthma in people who do not respond to bronchodilators alone. Also used in creams to treat inflammatory skin disorders and to relieve and prevent symptoms of vasomotor and allergic rhinitis.
Side-effects: cough, nasal discomfort/irritation, hoarse voice, sore throat, nosebleed (with inhalers/nasal spray).

Bendroflumethiazide/bendrofluazide (thiazide diuretic)

Used to treat hypertension, cardiac failure and resistant oedema. Also reduces urinary calcium excretion and so decreases rate of recurrence in patients with recurrent renal stones.
Side-effects: hypokalaemia, dehydration, postural hypotension, gout and hyperglycaemia.

Benzylpenicillin (penicillin antibiotic)

See antibiotics in Drug Classes.

Calcitonin (salmon)/Salcatonin (hormone)

Used to treat hypercalcaemia, bone pain in malignancy, osteoporosis and Paget's disease of bone.
Side-effects: nausea, vomiting, flushing.

Captopril (ACE inhibitor)

Reduces peripheral vasoconstriction and is used to treat hypertension, congestive heart failure, post-myocardial infarction and diabetic nephropathy.
Side-effects: postural hypotension, persistent dry cough, rash, loss of taste, reduced kidney function.

Carbamazepine (anticonvulsant)

Used to reduce likelihood of generalized tonic-clonic seizures and partial seizures. Also used to relieve severe pain in trigeminal neuralgia and for prophylaxis of bipolar disorder.
Side-effects: drowsiness, ataxia, blurred vision, confusion, nausea, loss of appetite.

Cefaclor (cephalosporin antibiotic)

See antibiotics in Drug Classes.

Cefotaxime (cephalosporin antibiotic)

See antibiotics in Drug Classes.

Cefuroxime (cephalosporin antibiotic)

See antibiotics in Drug Classes.

Chlorpromazine hydrochloride (antipsychotic)

Has a sedative effect and is used to control the symptoms of schizophrenia and to treat agitation without causing confusion and stupor. Also used to treat nausea and vomiting in terminally-ill patients.
Side-effects: extrapyramidal symptoms (e.g. parkinsonian symptoms, dystonia, akathisia, tardive dyskinesia), neuroleptic malignant syndrome, hypotension, dry mouth, blurred vision, urinary retention, constipation, jaundice.

Ciclosporin (immunosuppressant)

Used to prevent rejection of organ and tissue transplantation. Also used to treat rheumatoid arthritis, and severe resistant psoriasis and dermatitis when other treatments have failed.
Side-effects: nephrotoxicity, hypertension, increased body hair, nausea, tremor, swelling of gums.

Cimetidine (anti-ulcer – H_2-receptor antagonist)

Decreases gastric acid production and is used to treat gastric and duodenal ulcers, and for gastro-oesophageal reflux disease.
Side-effects: none.

Ciprofloxacin (antibacterial)

Treats mainly Gram negative infection and some Gram positive infections. Used for chest, intestine and urinary tract infections and to treat gonorrhoea.
Side-effects: nausea, vomiting, abdominal pain, diarrhoea.

Co-proxamol (compound analgesic)

Combination of a non-opioid and a mild opioid analgesic (paracetamol and dextropropoxyphene). Used to treat mild to moderate pain.
Side-effects: dizziness, drowsiness, nausea, vomiting, constipation. Dangerous in overdose.

Dexamethasone (glucocorticoid)

Suppresses inflammatory and allergic disorders. Used to diagnose Cushing's disease. Used to treat cerebral oedema, congenital adrenal hyperplasia, nausea and vomiting associated with chemotherapy and various types of shock.
Side-effects: indigestion, acne, increased body hair, moon-face, hypertension, weight gain/oedema, impaired glucose tolerance, cataract, glaucoma, osteoporosis, peptic ulcer, candida.

Diazepam (benzodiazepine)

Has a wide range of uses. Most commonly used to reduce anxiety, relax muscles, promote sleep and in the treatment of alcohol withdrawal. Also used for febrile convulsions and status epilepticus.

Side-effects: daytime drowsiness, dizziness, unsteadiness, confusion in the elderly. Dependence develops with prolonged use.

Diclofenac (non-steroidal anti-inflammatory)

Used to relieve mild to moderate pain associated with inflammation such as rheumatoid arthritis, osteoarthritis and musculoskeletal disorders. Also used to treat acute gout and postoperative pain.
Side-effects: gastrointestinal disorders.

Digoxin (cardiac glycoside)

Used in heart failure to control breathlessness, tiredness and fluid retention. Also used to treat supraventricular arrhythmias, particularly atrial fibrillation.
Side-effects: anorexia, nausea, vomiting, diarrhoea, visual disturbances, headache, tiredness, palpitations.

Dihydrocodeine/DF118 (opioid analgesic)

Used to relieve moderate acute and chronic pain.
Side-effects: drowsiness, nausea, vomiting, constipation, dizziness, dry mouth.

Diltiazem (calcium channel blocker)

Used to prevent and treat angina and to lower high blood pressure.
Side-effects: bradycardia, headache, nausea, dizziness, dry mouth, hypotension, ankle and leg swelling.

Dobutamine (inotropic sympathomimetic)

Provides inotropic support in acute severe heart failure, cardiac surgery, cardiomyopathies, septic shock and cardiogenic shock.
Common side-effect: tachycardias.

Dopamine (inotropic sympathomimetic)

Used to treat cardiogenic shock after myocardial infarction, hypotension after cardiac surgery, acute severe heart failure and to start diuresis in chronic heart failure.
Side-effects: nausea, vomiting, peripheral vasoconstriction, hypotension, hypertension, tachycardia.

Doxapram (respiratory stimulant)

Used in hospital under expert supervision to treat acute exacerbations of COPD with type II respiratory failure when ventilation is unavailable or contraindicated.
Side-effects: tachycardia, hypertension, cerebral oedema, hyperthyroidism, dizziness, sweating, confusion, seizures, nausea, vomiting, perineal warmth.

Epinephrine/adrenaline (sympathomimetic agent)

See Adrenaline.

Erythromycin (macrolide antibiotic)

See antibiotics in Drug Classes.

Fentanyl (opioid analgesic)

Used to depress respiration in patients needing prolonged assisted ventilation. Also used as an analgesic during surgery and to enhance anaesthesia.
Side-effects: drowsiness, nausea, vomiting, constipation, dizziness, dry mouth.

Ferrous sulphate (iron salt)

Used to treat iron-deficiency anaemia.
Side-effects: nausea, epigastric pain, constipation or diarrhoea, darkening of faeces.

Flucloxacillin (penicillin antibiotic)

See antibiotics in Drug Classes.

Fluoxetine (selective serotonin re-uptake inhibitor)

More commonly known by its brand name, Prozac, it increases serotonin levels and is used to treat depressive illness, obsessive–compulsive disorder and bulimia nervosa.
Side-effects: headache, nervousness, insomnia, anxiety, nausea, diarrhoea, weight loss, sexual dysfunction.

Furosemide/frusemide (loop diuretic)

A powerful, fast-acting diuretic that is used in emergencies to reduce acute pulmonary oedema secondary to left ventricular failure. It also reduces oedema and dyspnoea associated

with chronic heart failure and is used to treat oliguria secondary to acute renal failure.
Side-effects: postural hypotension, hypokalaemia, hyponatraemia, hyperuricaemia, gout, dizziness, nausea.

Gentamicin (aminoglycoside antibiotic)

See antibiotics in Drug Classes.

Gliclazide (sulphonylurea)

Oral antidiabetic drug that lowers blood sugar and is used to treat type II diabetes mellitus.
Side-effects: hyperglycaemia, weight gain.

GTN/glyceryl trinitrate (organic nitrate)

A potent coronary and peripheral vasodilator that relieves angina and is used to treat heart failure.
Side-effects: headaches, dizziness, flushing, postural hypotension, tachycardias.

Haloperidol (butyrophenone)

Used to control violent and dangerously impulsive behaviour associated with psychotic disorders such as schizophrenia, mania and dementia. Also used to treat motor tics.
Side-effects: Parkinsonism, acute dystonia, akathisia, drowsiness, postural hypotension.

Heparin (anticoagulant)

Prevents blood clots forming and is used to prevent and treat deep vein thrombosis and pulmonary embolism. Also used in the management of unstable angina, myocardial infarction and acute occlusion of peripheral arteries.
Side-effects: haemorrhage, thrombocytopenia.

Hydrocortisone (glucocorticoid)

Given as replacement therapy for adrenocortical insufficiency. Suppresses a variety of inflammatory and allergic disorders, e.g. psoriasis, eczema, rheumatic disease, inflammatory bowel disease. Also used as an immunosuppressant following organ transplant and for treating shock.

Side-effects: indigestion, acne, increased body hair, moon-face, hypertension, weight gain/oedema, impaired glucose tolerance, cataract, glaucoma, osteoporosis, peptic ulcer, candida.

Hyoscine (muscarinic antagonist)

Used to manage motion sickness, giddiness and nausea caused by disturbances of the inner ear and reduce intestinal spasm in irritable bowel syndrome. Used as a pre-medication to dry bronchial secretions before surgery.
Side-effects: sedation, dry mouth, blurred vision.

Ibuprofen (non-steroidal anti-inflammatory)

Used to reduce pain, stiffness and inflammation associated with conditions such as rheumatoid arthritis, osteoarthritis, sprains and other soft tissue injuries. Also used to treat post-operative pain, headache, migraine, menstrual and dental pain, and fever and pain in children.
Side-effects: heartburn, indigestion.

Insulin (peptide hormone)

Lowers blood sugar and is given by injection to control type I (insulin-dependent) and sometimes type II (maturity-onset) diabetes mellitus.
Side-effects: injection site irritation, weakness, sweating, hypoglycaemia, weight gain.

Interferon (antiviral and anticancer)

Group of proteins produced by the body in response to viral infection that stimulate the immune response:

Interferon alfa – used for certain lymphomas and tumours (e.g. leukaemia) and chronic active hepatitis B and C. *Side-effects*: anorexia, nausea, influenza-like symptoms, lethargy.

Interferon beta – used for relapses of multiple sclerosis. *Side-effects*: irritation at injection site, influenza-like symptoms.

Interferon gamma – used in conjunction with antibiotics to treat chronic granulomatous disease. *Side-effects*: fever, headache, chills, myalgia, fatigue, nausea, vomiting, arthralgia, rashes and injection-site reactions.

Ipratropium bromide (anticholinergic)

Bronchodilator that is used to treat reversible airways obstruction, particularly in chronic obstructive pulmonary disease. It is also prescribed as a nasal spray to treat runny nose due to allergy.
Side-effects: dry mouth and throat.

Isoprenaline (inotropic sympathomimetic)

Increases heart rate and cardiac contractility. Used to treat heart block and severe bradycardia.
Side-effects: tachycardia, arrhythmias, hypotension, sweating, tremor, headache.

Isosorbide mononitrate (organic nitrate)

A coronary and peripheral vasodilator. Used as a prophylaxis in angina and as an adjunct in congestive heart failure.
Side-effects: headaches, dizziness, flushing, postural hypotension, tachycardias.

Ketamine (intravenous anaesthetic)

Used to induce and maintain anaesthesia during surgery.
Side-effects: hallucinations and other transient psychotic sequelae, increased blood pressure, tachycardia, increased muscle tone, apnoea, hypotension.

Lactulose (osmotic laxative)

Used to relieve constipation. Also used to treat hepatic encephalopathy.
Side-effects: flatulence, belching, stomach cramps, diarrhoea.

Levodopa/L-dopa (dopamine precursor)

Used to treat idiopathic Parkinson's disease by replacing the depleted dopamine in the brain. It is combined with an inhibitor such as carbidopa (to form co-caraldopa) or benserazide (to form co-beneldopa) which prolongs and enhances its action. It becomes less effective with continued use.
Side-effects: nausea, vomiting, abdominal pain, anorexia, postural hypotension, dysrhythmias, dizziness, discoloration of urine and other bodily fluids, abnormal involuntary movements, nervousness, agitation.

Lidocaine/lignocaine (local anaesthetic, class I anti-arrhythmic agent)

Used as a local anaesthetic and for ventricular dysrhythmias, especially following myocardial infarction.
Side-effects: nausea, vomiting, drowsiness, dizziness.

Lisinopril (ACE inhibitor)

Vasodilator that is used to treat hypertension, congestive heart failure and following myocardial infarction.
Side-effects: nausea, vomiting, dry cough, altered sense of taste, hypotension.

Lithium (antimanic)

Used to prevent and treat mania, bipolar disorders and recurrent depression. Its effects (including toxicity) are increased if it is combined with a thiazide diuretic.
Side-effects: weight gain, nausea, vomiting, diarrhoea, fine tremor.

Loperamide (antimotility)

Inhibits peristalsis and prevents the loss of water and electrolytes. Used to treat diarrhoea.
Side-effects: none.

Mannitol (osmotic diuretic)

Reduces cerebral oedema and therefore intracranial pressure. Used preoperatively to reduce intraocular pressure in glaucoma.
Side-effects: chills, fever, fluid/electrolyte imbalance.

Metformin (biguanide)

Used to treat type II diabetes mellitus by decreasing glucose production, increasing peripheral glucose utilization and reducing glucose absorption in the digestive tract.
Side-effects: anorexia, nausea, vomiting, diarrhoea.

Methotrexate (cytotoxic and immunosuppressive)

Inhibits DNA, RNA and protein synthesis leading to cell death. Used to treat leukaemia, lymphoma and a number of solid tumours. Also used for rheumatoid arthritis and psoriasis.

Side-effects: bone marrow suppression, anorexia, diarrhoea, nausea, vomiting, hepatotoxicity, dry cough, mouth and gum ulcers and inflammation.

Methyldopa (antihypertensive)

Used to treat high blood pressure, especially in pregnancy.
Side-effects: drowsiness, headache, postural hypotension, depression, impotence.

Metoclopramide (dopamine antagonist)

Used to treat nausea and vomiting caused by radiotherapy, anti-cancer drug and opioid treatment, migraines, and following surgery. Also used to reduce symptoms of gastro-oesophageal reflux.
Side-effects: acute dystonic reactions especially in children and young adults.

Midazolam (benzodiazepine)

Water-soluble and short acting, it is given by injection or infusion to relieve anxiety and to provide sedation with amnesia. Used during small procedures under local anaesthetic and in ITU units for those on ventilatory support.
Side-effects: apnoea, hypotension, drowsiness, lightheadedness, confusion, ataxia, amnesia, dependence, muscle weakness.

Milrinone (phosphodiesterase inhibitor)

A positive inotrope with vasodilating properties, it increases cardiac contractility and reduces vascular resistance. Used to treat severe congestive heart failure and myocardial dysfunction.
Side-effects: hypotension, cardiac arrhythmias, tachycardia, headache, insomnia, nausea, vomiting, diarrhoea.

Morphine (opioid analgesic)

Used to relieve severe pain and suppress cough in palliative care. Also effective in the relief of acute left ventricular failure.
Side-effects: drowsiness, nausea, vomiting, constipation, dizziness, dry mouth and respiratory depression.

Naloxone (antagonist for central and respiratory depression)

Used to reverse respiratory depression caused by opioid analgesics, mainly in overdose.
Side-effects: nausea, vomiting, tachycardia, fibrillation.

Nifedipine (calcium channel blocker)

Used to treat hypertension, angina and Raynaud's disease.
Side-effects: headache, flushing, ankle swelling, dizziness, fatigue, hypotension.

Nimodipine (calcium channel blocker)

Relaxes vascular smooth muscle, acting preferentially on the cerebral arteries. Used to treat cerebral vasospasm associated with subarachnoid haemorrhage.
Side-effects: hypotension, ECG abnormalities, headache, gastrointestinal disorders, nausea, sweating.

Nitrous oxide (inhalational agent)

Used for maintenance of anaesthesia and, in smaller doses, for analgesia without loss of consciousness, especially in labour.
Side-effects are rare.

Noradrenaline/norepinephrine (sympathomimetic agent)

Administered intravenously to constrict peripheral vessels to raise blood pressure in patients with acute hypotension.
Side-effects: hypertension, headache, bradycardia, arrhythmias, peripheral ischaemia.

Omeprazole (proton-pump inhibitor)

Reduces the amount of acid produced by the stomach and is used to treat stomach and duodenal ulcers as well as gastro-oesophageal reflux and oesophagitis.
Side-effects: headache, diarrhoea.

Ondansetron (serotonin antagonist)

Used to treat nausea and vomiting associated with anticancer drug therapy, radiotherapy and following surgery.
Side-effects: headache, constipation.

Oxitropium bromide (anticholinergic)

Bronchodilator that is used to treat reversible airways obstruction, particularly in chronic obstructive pulmonary disease.
Side-effects: dry mouth and throat.

Oxytetracycline (tetracycline antibiotic)

See antibiotics in Drug Classes.

Pancuronium (muscle relaxant)

Long acting, it is used as a muscle relaxant during surgical procedures and to facilitate tracheal intubation. Also used on patients receiving long-term mechanical ventilation.
Side-effects: tachycardia, hypertension, skin flushing, hypotension, bronchospasm.

Paracetamol (non-opioid analgesic)

Used to treat mild pain and reduce fever. Does not irritate the gastric mucosa and so can be used by those who have peptic ulcers or can be used in place of aspirin for those who are aspirin-intolerant.
Side-effects are rare but overdose is dangerous, causing liver failure.

Pethidine (opioid analgesic)

Used to treat moderate to severe pain, especially during labour.
Side-effects: dizziness, nausea, vomiting, drowsiness, confusion, constipation.

Phenytoin (anticonvulsant)

Used to treat all forms of epilepsy (except absence seizures) as well as trigeminal neuralgia.
Side-effects: dizziness, headache, confusion, nausea, vomiting, insomnia, acne, increased body hair.

Prednisolone (glucocorticoid)

In high doses it is used to suppress inflammatory and allergic disorders e.g. asthma, eczema, inflammatory bowel disease, rheumatoid arthritis. Also used as an immunosuppressant following organ transplant and to treat leukaemia. It is used

in lower doses for replacement therapy in adrenal deficiency, though cortisol (hydrocortisone) is preferred.
Side-effects: indigestion, acne, increased body hair, moon-face, hypertension, weight gain/oedema, impaired glucose tolerance, cataract, glaucoma, osteoporosis, peptic ulcer, candida, adrenal suppression.

Propofol (i.v. anaesthetic)
Used to induce and maintain anaesthesia. Also used as a sedative on ITU and during investigative procedures.
Side-effects: hypotension, tremor.

Ramipril (ACE inhibitor)
As a vasodilator it is used to treat hypertension and congestive heart failure. Also used following myocardial infarction.
Side-effects: nausea, dizziness, headache, cough, dry mouth, taste disturbance.

Rifampicin (antituberculous agent)
Antibacterial used to treat tuberculosis, leprosy and other serious infections such as Legionnaire's disease and osteomyelitis. Used as a prophylactic against menigococcal meningitis and *Haemophilus influenzae* (type b) infection.
Side-effects: red-orange coloured tears and urine.

Salbutamol (β_2 agonist)
A bronchodilator, it is used to relieve asthma, chronic bronchitis and emphysema. It is also used in premature labour to relax uterine muscle.
Side-effects: tremor, tachycardia, anxiety, nervous tension, restlessness.

Salcatonin
See calcitonin.

Salmeterol (β_2 agonist)
A bronchodilator that is used to treat asthma and bronchospasms. It is longer acting than salbutamol and so is useful

in preventing nocturnal asthma. It should not be used to relieve acute asthma attacks as it has a slow onset of effect.
Side-effects: fine tremors, especially in the hands.

Senna (stimulant laxative)

Used to treat constipation by increasing the response of the colon to normal stimuli.
Side-effects: abdominal cramps, diarrhoea.

Simvastatin (HMG CoA reductase inhibitor)

Lowers LDL cholesterol and is prescribed for people who have not responded to diet modification to protect them from cardiovascular disease.
Side-effects: none.

Sodium cromoglicate (mast cell inhibitor)

Used to prevent the onset of asthma and other allergic conditions. It has a slow onset of action and so is not useful in treating acute asthma. It is also used to prevent allergic conjunctivitis, allergic rhinitis and for food allergies.
Side-effects: cough, hoarseness, throat irritation, bronchospasm.

Sodium valproate (antiepileptic)

Used to treat all types of epilepsy.
Side-effects: nausea, vomiting, weight gain. Administered with care in pregnancy.

Streptokinase (fibrinolytic agent)

An enzyme that dissolves blood clots by acting on the fibrin contained within it. Due to its fast acting nature it is useful in treating acute myocardial infarction. Also used to treat a number of thromboembolic events such as pulmonary embolism and thrombosed arteriovenous shunts.
Side-effects: excessive bleeding, hypotension, nausea, vomiting, allergic reactions.

Sulfasalazine (aminosalicylate)

Used as an anti-inflammatory to treat ulcerative colitis and active Crohn's disease. Also found to help in the treatment of rheumatoid arthritis.

Side-effects: nausea, vomiting, loss of appetite, headache, joint pain, abdominal discomfort, anorexia.

Sumatriptan (serotonin agonist)

Used to treat acute migraine and cluster headaches.
Side-effects: pain at injection site, feeling of tingling/heat, flushing, feeling of heaviness/weakness, lethargy.

Temazepam (benzodiazepine)

Used as a short-term treatment for insomnia and as a premedication before surgery.
Side-effects: daytime drowsiness, dependence.

Terbutaline (β_2 agonist)

Acts as a bronchodilator and is used to treat and prevent bronchospasm associated with asthma, chronic bronchitis and emphysema.
Side-effects: nausea, vomiting, fine tremor, restlessness, anxiety.

Tetracycline (tetracycline antibiotic)

See antibiotics in Drug Classes.

Theophylline (methylxanthine)

Acts as a bronchodilator and is used to treat asthma, bronchitis and emphysema.
Side-effects: headache, nausea, vomiting, palpitations.

Thiopental (barbiturate)

Used to induce general anaesthesia, as well as reducing intracranial pressure in patients whose ventilation is controlled.
Side-effects: cardiovascular and respiratory depression.

Tramadol (opioid analgesic)

Used to treat moderate to severe pain.
Side-effects: nausea, vomiting, dry mouth, tiredness, drowsiness, dependence.

Vecuronium (muscle relaxant)

Used as a muscle relaxant during surgical procedures and to facilitate tracheal intubation, it has an intermediate duration of action.
Side-effects: skin flushing, hypotension, bronchospasm are rare.

Verapamil (calcium channel blocker)

Used in the treatment of hypertension, angina and supraventricular dysrhythmias.
Side-effects: constipation, headache, ankle swelling, nausea, vomiting.

Warfarin (oral anticoagulant)

Prevention and treatment of pulmonary embolism and deep vein thrombosis. Decreases the risk of transient ischaemic attacks as well as thromboembolism in people with atrial fibrillation and following artificial heart valve surgery.
Side-effects: haemorrhage, bruising.

Bronchodilator brand names

Aminophylline	Amnivent, Phyllocontin
Beclometasone	Aerobec, Beclazone, Becloforte, Becodisks, Beconase, Becotide,
Ipratropium bromide	Atrovent, Rinatec, Respontin
Oxitropium	Oxivent
Salbutamol	Aerolin, Airomir, Asmasal, Salamol, Salbulin, Ventmax, Ventodisks, Ventolin, Volmax
Salmeterol	Serevent
Terbutaline	Bricanyl, Monovent
Theophylline	Lasma, Nuelin, Theo-Dur, Uniphyllin

Prescription abbreviations

Abbreviation	Latin	English
a.c.	*ante cibum*	before food
ad lib	*ad libitum*	as desired
b.d.	*bis die*	twice a day
o.d.	*omni die*	daily
o.m.	*omni mane*	in the mornings
o.n.	*omni nocte*	at night
p.c.	*post cibum*	after food
p.r.n.	*pro re nata*	when required
q.d.s.	*quater die sumendus*	four times a day
q.q.h.	*quarta quaque hora*	every four hours
stat.	*statim*	immediately
t.d.s.	*ter die sumendus*	three times a day

Further reading

BMA/RPSGB 2002 British National Formulary, 44th edn. British Medical Association and Royal Pharmaceutical Society of Great Britain, London

Chatu S, Milson A, Tofield C 2000 Hands-on guide to clinical pharmacology. Blackwell Science, Oxford

Henry J A 2001 New guide to medicine and drugs, 5th edn. British Medical Association, London

Ritter J, Lewis L D, Mant T G K 1999 A textbook of clinical pharmacology, 4th edn. Arnold, London

Zaloga G P, MacGregor D 1997 The critical care drug handbook, 2nd edn. Mosby, St Louis

SECTION 5

Appendices

Electrotherapy (Kitchen 2002, with permission)

Contraindications and precautions for electrotherapy modalities are constantly being reviewed as continuing research gives us a better understanding of the effects and consequences of treatment. In some instances the evidence for some of the contraindications/precautions is not conclusive. However, where there is a remote chance that the modality may cause an adverse effect this has been highlighted. All patients are different and we need to use our clinical judgement to weigh up the benefits of electrotherapy against the potential hazards.

Ultrasound

Potential hazards

Do not apply over the following:

- Uterus during pregnancy
- Gonads
- Malignancies and precancerous lesions
- Tissues previously treated by deep X-ray or other radiation
- Vascular abnormalities, e.g. deep vein thrombosis, emboli, severe atherosclerosis
- Acute infections
- Cardiac area in advanced heart disease
- Eye
- Stellate ganglion
- Haemophiliacs not covered by factor replacement
- Areas over subcutaneous bony prominences
- Epiphyseal plates
- Spinal cord after laminectomy
- Subcutaneous major nerves
- Cranium
- Anaesthetic areas

Interferential

Contraindications

- Patients where disturbance of a thrombus, spread of infection or cancerous cell haemorrhage might result
- Pacemakers
- Abdomen during pregnancy
- Chest wall in patients with cardiac problems

Short-wave diathermy

Contraindications

- Implanted pacemakers
- Metal in the tissues or external fixators
- Impaired thermal sensations
- Uncooperative patients
- Pregnancy
- Haemorrhaging areas
- Ischaemic tissue
- Malignant tumours
- Active tuberculosis
- Recent venous thrombosis
- Patient pyrexia
- Areas of skin affected by course of X-ray

Growing epiphysis should be treated with caution.

Transcutaneous electrical nerve stimulation (TENS)

Contraindications (unless recommended by a medical practitioner)

- Undiagnosed pain
- Pacemakers
- Heart disease
- Epilepsy

- Pregnancy
  - first trimester
  - over the uterus

Do not apply TENS over:

- The carotid sinus (anterior neck)
- On broken skin
- On dysaesthetic skin
- Internally (mouth)

Low-intensity laser therapy

Contraindications

- Direct treatment of the eye
- In patients with active or suspected carcinoma
- Direct irradiation over the pregnant uterus
- Areas of haemorrhage
- Cognitive difficulties or unreliable patient

Other safety considerations

Exercise caution when treating the following:

- Infected tissue such as an infected open wound
- The sympathetic ganglia, vagus nerves and cardiac region in patients with heart disease
- Photosensitive areas
- Patients with epilepsy
- Areas of altered skin sensation

Neuromuscular electrical stimulation (NMES)

Contraindications

- Pacemakers
- Peripheral vascular disease
- Hypertensive and hypotensive subjects
- Areas of excessive adipose tissue in obese subjects
- Neoplastic tissue

- Areas of active tissue infection
- Devitalized skin, e.g. post deep X-ray therapy
- Patients with a reduced understanding of the intervention or ability to provide feedback during treatment

Do not apply over the following:

- Carotid sinus
- Thoracic region
- Phrenic nerve
- Trunk, in a pregnant subject

Heat

Contraindications

- Lack of local thermal sensitivity on the part of the patient
- Impaired circulation
- Areas of recent bleeding or haemorrhaging
- Devitalized skin, e.g. after deep X-ray treatment
- Open wounds
- Certain skin conditions, e.g. skin carcinomas, acute dermatitis
- Cardiovascular impairment
- Damaged or infected tissue

Cold (cryotherapy)

Contraindications

- Arteriosclerosis
- Peripheral vascular disease
- Vasospasm
- Cryoglobinaemia
- Cold urticaria

Caution should also be exercised with patients who have:

- **Cardiac disease and altered arterial blood pressure**
- **Defective skin sensation**

- Skin hypersensitivity
- Adverse psychological factors

Care should also be taken when treating areas in which nervous tissue is very superficial.

Infrared irradiation

Contraindications

- Areas with poor or deficient cutaneous thermal sensitivity
- Subjects with advanced cardiovascular disease
- Local areas of impaired peripheral circulation
- Scar tissue or tissue devitalized by deep X-ray treatment or other ionizing radiation
- Malignant tissue of the skin
- Subjects with a reduced level of consciousness or understanding of the dangers of treatment
- Subjects with acute febrile illness
- Some acute skin diseases, e.g. dermatitis, eczema
- The testes

Reference

Kitchen S 2002 Electrotherapy: evidence-based practice, 11th edn. Churchill Livingstone, Edinburgh

Abbreviations

AAA	abdominal aortic aneurysm
Ab	antibody
ABGs	arterial blood gases
ABPA	allergic bronchopulmonary aspergillosis
ACBT	active cycle of breathing technique
ACE	angiotensin converting enzyme
ACT	activated clotting time
ACTH	adrenocorticotrophic hormone

AD	autogenic drainage
ADH	anti-diuretic hormone
ADL	activities of daily living
ADR	adverse drug reaction
AE	air entry
AEA	above elbow amputation
AF	atrial fibrillation
AFB	acid fast bacillus
AFO	ankle foot orthosis
Ag	antigen
AGN	acute glomerulonephritis
AHRF	acute hypoxaemic respiratory failure
AI	aortic insufficiency
AIDS	acquired immune deficiency syndrome
AKA	above knee amputation
AL	acute leukaemia
ALD	alcoholic liver disease
ALI	acute lung injury
AML	acute myeloid leukaemia
AP	anteroposterior
APACHE	acute physiology and chronic health evaluation
ARDS	acute respiratory distress syndrome
ARF	acute renal failure
AROM	active range of movement
AS	ankylosing spondylitis
ASD	atrial septal defect
ATN	acute tubular necrosis
AVAS	absolute visual analogue scale
AVF	arteriovenous fistula
AVR	aortic valve replacement
AVSD	atrioventricular septal defect
AXR	abdominal X-ray
BE	bacterial endocarditis/barium enema/base excess
BEA	below elbow amputation
BiPAP	bilevel positive airway pressure
BIVAD	biventricular device

BKA	below knee amputation
BM	blood glucose monitoring
BMI	body mass index
BO	bowels open
BP	blood pressure
BPD	bronchopulmonary dysplasia
BPF	bronchopleural fistula
bpm	beats per minute
BS	bowel sounds/breath sounds
BSA	body surface area
BSO	bilateral salpingo-oophorectomy
BVHF	bi-ventricular heart failure
Ca	carcinoma
CABG	coronary artery bypass graft
CAD	coronary artery disease
CAH	chronic active hepatitis
CAL	chronic airflow limitation
CAO	chronic airways obstruction
CAPD	continuous ambulatory peritoneal dialysis
CAVG	coronary artery vein graft
CAVHF	continuous arterial venous haemofiltration
CBD	common bile duct
CBF	cerebral blood flow
CCF	congestive cardiac failure
CCU	coronary care unit
CDH	congenital dislocation of the hip
CF	cystic fibrosis
CFA	cryptogenic fibrosing alveolitis
CHD	coronary heart disease
CHF	chronic heart failure
CI	chest infection
CK	creatine kinase
CLD	chronic lung disease
CML	chronic myeloid leukaemia
CMV	controlled mandatory ventilation/ cytomegalovirus

CNS	central nervous system
CO	cardiac output
C/O	complains of
COAD	chronic obstructive airways disease
COPD	chronic obstructive pulmonary disease
CP	cerebral palsy
CPAP	continuous positive airway pressure
CPM	continuous passive movements
CPN	community psychiatric nurse
CPP	cerebral perfusion pressure
CPR	cardiopulmonary resuscitation
CRF	chronic renal failure
CRP	C-reactive protein
CSF	cerebrospinal fluid
CT	computed tomography
CTEV	congenital talipes equinovarus
CV	closing volume
CVA	cerebrovascular accident
CVP	central venous pressure
CVS	cardiovascular system
CVVHF	continuous veno-venous haemofiltration
CXR	chest X-ray
D&C	dilation and curettage
D/C	discharge
D/W	discussed with
DBE	deep breathing exercises
DDH	developmental dysplasia of the hips
DH	drug history
DHS	dynamic hip screw
DIB	difficulty in breathing
DIC	disseminated intravascular coagulopathy
DIOS	distal intestinal obstruction syndrome
DLCO	diffusing capacity for carbon monoxide
DM	diabetes mellitus
DMD	Duchenne muscular dystrophy
DN	district nurse

DNA	deoxyribonucleic acid/did not attend
DSA	digital subtraction angiography
DU	duodenal ulcer
DVT	deep vein thrombosis
DXT	deep X-ray therapy
EBV	Epstein–Barr virus
ECG	electrocardiogram
EEG	electroencephalogram
EIA	exercise-induced asthma
EMG	electromyography
ENT	ear, nose and throat
EOR	end of range
Ep	epilepsy
EPAP	expiratory positive airway pressure
EPP	equal pressure points
ERCP	endoscopic retrograde cholangiopancreatography
ERV	expiratory reserve volume
ESR	erythrocyte sedimentation rate
ESRF	end stage renal failure
$ETCO_2$	end-tidal carbon dioxide
ETT	endotracheal tube
EUA	examination under anaesthetic
FB	foreign body
FBC	full blood count
FDP	fibrin degradation product
FET	forced expiration technique
FEV_1	forced expiratory volume in 1 second
FFD	fixed flexion deformity
FG	French gauge
FGF	fibroblast growth factor
FH	family history
FHF	fulminant hepatic failure
FiO_2	fractional inspired oxygen concentration
FRC	functional residual capacity
FROM	full range of movement

FVC	forced vital capacity
FWB	full weight bearing
GA	general anaesthetic
GBS	Guillain–Barré syndrome
GCS	Glasgow Coma Scale
GH	general health
GIT	gastrointestinal tract
GOR	gastro-oesophageal reflux
GPB	glossopharyngeal breathing
GTN	glycerol trinitrate
GU	gastric ulcer/genitourinary
H^+	hydrogen ion
$[H^+]$	hydrogen ion concentration
HASO	hip abduction spinal orthosis
Hb	haemoglobin
HC	head circumference
Hct	haematocrit
HD	haemodialysis
HDU	high dependency unit
HF	heart failure
HFCWO	high-frequency chest wall oscillation
HFJV	high-frequency jet ventilation
HFO	high-frequency oscillation
HFOV	high-frequency oscillatory ventilation
HFPPV	high-frequency positive pressure ventilation
HH	hiatus hernia/home help
HI	head injury
HIV	human immunodeficiency virus
HLA	human leucocyte antigen
HLT	heart–lung transplantation
HME	heat and moisture exchanger
HPC	history of presenting condition
HPOA	hypertrophic pulmonary osteoarthropathy
HR	heart rate
HRR	heart rate reserve
HT	hypertension

IABP	intra-aortic balloon pump
ICC	intercostal catheter
ICD	intercostal drain
ICP	intracranial pressure
ICU	intensive care unit
IDC	indwelling catheter
IDDM	insulin dependent diabetes mellitus
Ig	immunoglobulin
IHD	ischaemic heart disease
ILD	interstitial lung disease
IM	intramedullary
IM/i.m.	intramuscular
IMA	internal mammary artery
IMV	intermittent mandatory ventilation
INR	international normalized ratio
IPAP	inspiratory positive airway pressure
IPPB	intermittent positive pressure breathing
IPPV	intermittent positive pressure ventilation
IPS	inspiratory pressure support
IRV	inspiratory reserve volume
IS	incentive spirometry
ITU	intensive therapy unit
IV/i.v.	intravenous
IVB	intervertebral block
IVC	inferior vena cava
IVH	intraventricular haemorrhage
IVI	intravenous infusion
IVOX	intravenacaval oxygenation
IVUS	intravascular ultrasound
JVP	jugular venous pressure
KAFO	knee ankle foot orthosis
KO	knee orthosis
LA	local anaesthetic
LAP	left atrial pressure
LBBB	left bundle branch block
LBP	low back pain

LED	light-emitting diode
LFT	liver function test/lung function test
LL	lower limb/lower lobe
LOC	level of consciousness
LP	lumbar puncture
LRTD	lower respiratory tract disease
LSCS	lower segment caesarean section
LTOT	long-term oxygen therapy
LVAD	left ventricular assist device
LVEF	left ventricular ejection fraction
LVF	left ventricular failure
LVRS	lung volume reduction surgery
MAP	mean airway pressure/mean arterial pressure
MAS	minimal access surgery
MCH	mean corpuscular haemoglobin
MC&S	microbiology, culture and sensitivity
MCV	mean corpuscular volume
MDI	metered dose inhaler
ME	metabolic equivalents/myalgic encephalomyelitis
MI	myocardial infarction
ML	middle lobe
MM	muscle
MMAD	mass median aerodynamic diameter
MND	motor neurone disease
MOW	meals on wheels
MRI	magnetic resonance imaging
MRSA	methicillin-resistant *Staphylococcus aureus*
MS	mitral stenosis/multiple sclerosis
MSU	midstream urine
MUA	manipulation under anaesthetic
MVO_2	myocardial oxygen consumption
MVR	mitral valve replacement
MVV	maximum voluntary ventilation
NAD	nothing abnormal detected
NAI	non-accidental injury

NBI	no bony injury
NBL	non-directed bronchial lavage
NBM	nil by mouth
NCPAP	nasal continuous positive airway pressure
NEPV	negative extrathoracic pressure ventilation
NFR	not for resuscitation
NG	nasogastric
NH	nursing home
NIDDM	non-insulin dependent diabetes mellitus
NIPPV	non-invasive intermittent positive pressure ventilation
NITU	neonatal intensive care unit
NIV	non-invasive ventilation
NOF	neck of femur
NOH	neck of humerus
NP	nasopharyngeal
NPA	nasopharyngeal airway
NPV	negative pressure ventilation
NR	nodal rhythm
NREM	non-rapid eye movement
N/S	nursing staff
NSAID	non-steroidal anti-inflammatory drug
NSR	normal sinus rhythm
NWB	non-weight bearing
OA	oral airway/osteoarthritis
OB	obliterative bronchiolitis
OD	overdose
O/E	on examination
OGD	oesophagogastroduodenoscopy
OHFO	oral high-frequency oscillation
OI	oxygen index
OLT	orthotopic liver transplantation
OPD	outpatient department
ORIF	open reduction and internal fixation
OT	occupational therapist

PA	pernicious anaemia/posteroanterior/ pulmonary artery
P_ACO_2	partial pressure of carbon dioxide in alveolar gas
$PaCO_2$	partial pressure of carbon dioxide in arterial blood
PADL	personal activities of daily living
P_AO_2	partial pressure of oxygen in alveolar gas
PaO_2	partial pressure of oxygen in arterial blood
PAP	pulmonary artery pressure
PAWP	pulmonary artery wedge pressure
PBC	primary biliary cirrhosis
PC	presenting condition/pressure control
PCA	patient-controlled analgesia
PCD	primary ciliary dyskinesia
PCIRV	pressure-controlled inverse ratio ventilation
PCP	*Pneumocystis carinii* pneumonia
PCPAP	periodic continuous positive airway pressure
PCV	packed cell volume
PCWP	pulmonary capillary wedge pressure
PD	Parkinson's disease/peritoneal dialysis/ postural drainage
PDA	patent ductus arteriosus
PE	pulmonary embolus
PEEP	positive end-expiratory pressure
PEF	peak expiratory flow
PEFR	peak expiratory flow rate
PEG	percutaneous endoscopic gastrostomy
PeMax	peak expiratory mouth pressure
PEP	positive expiratory pressure
PFC	persistent foetal circulation
PFO	persistent foramen ovale
PHC	pulmonary hypertension crisis
PID	pelvic inflammatory disease
PIE	pulmonary interstitial emphysema
PIF	peak inspiratory flow

PIFR	peak inspiratory flow rate
***Pi*Max**	peak inspiratory mouth pressure
PIP	peak inspiratory pressure
PMH	previous medical history
PMR	percutaneous myocardial revascularization
PN	percussion note
PND	paroxysmal nocturnal dyspnoea
POMR	problem oriented medical record
POP	plaster of paris
PROM	passive range of movement
PS	pressure support/pulmonary stenosis
PTB	pulmonary tuberculosis
PTCA	percutaneous transluminal coronary angioplasty
PTFE	polytetrafluoroethylene
PTT	partial thromboplastin time
PVC	polyvinyl chloride
PVD	peripheral vascular disease
PVH	periventricular haemorrhage
PVL	periventricular leucomalacia
PVR	pulmonary vascular resistance
PWB	partial weight bearing
QOL	quality-of-life
RA	rheumatoid arthritis/room air
RAP	right atrial pressure
RBBB	right bundle branch block
RBC	red blood cell
RDS	respiratory distress syndrome
REM	rapid eye movement
RFT	respiratory function test
RH	residential home
RhF	rheumatic fever
RIP	rest in peace
RMT	respiratory muscle training
R/O	removal of
ROM	range of movement

ROP	retinopathy of prematurity
RPE	rating of perceived exertion
RPP	rate pressure product
RR	respiratory rate
RS	respiratory system
RSV	respiratory syncytial virus
RTA	road traffic accident
RV	residual volume
RVF	right ventricular failure
SA	sinoatrial
SAH	subarachnoid haemorrhage
SALT	speech and language therapist
SaO_2	arterial oxygen saturation
SB	sinus bradycardia
SBE	subacute bacterial endocarditis
SCI	spinal cord injury
SDH	subdural haematoma
SG_{AW}	specific airway conductance
SH	social history
SHO	senior house officer
SIMV	synchronized intermittent mandatory ventilation
SLAP	superior labrum, anterior and posterior
SLE	systemic lupus erythematosus
SMA	spinal muscle atrophy
SN	Swedish nose
SOA	swelling of ankles
SOB	shortness of breath
SOBAR	short of breath at rest
SOBOE	short of breath on exertion
SOOB	sit out of bed
SpO_2	pulse oximetry arterial oxygen saturation
SpR	special registrar
SPS	single point stick
SR	sinus rhythm
SS	social services

ST	sinus tachycardia
SV	self-ventilating
SVC	superior vena cava
SVD	spontaneous vaginal delivery
SVG	saphenous vein graft
SVO_2	mixed venous oxygen saturation
SVR	systemic vascular resistance
SVT	supra ventricular tachycardia
SW	social worker
T21	trisomy 21 (Down's syndrome)
TAA	thoracic aortic aneurysm
TAH	total abdominal hysterectomy
TAVR	tissue atrial valve repair
TB	tuberculosis
TBI	traumatic brain injury
$TcCO_2$	transcutaneous carbon dioxide
TcO_2	transcutaneous oxygen
TED	thromboembolic deterrent
TEE	thoracic expansion exercises
TENS	transcutaneous electrical nerve stimulation
TFA	transfemoral arteriogram
TGA	transposition of the great arteries
THR	total hip replacement
TIA	transient ischaemic attack
TKA	through knee amputation
TKR	total knee replacement
TLC	total lung capacity
TLCO	transfer factor in lung of carbon monoxide
TLSO	thoracolumbar spinal orthosis
TM	tracheostomy mask
TMR	transmyocardial revascularization
TMVR	tissue mitral valve repair
TOP	termination of pregnancy
TPN	total parenteral nutrition
TPR	temperature, pulse and respiration

TURBT	trans urethral resection of bladder tumour
TURP	trans urethral resection of prostate
TV	tidal volume
TWB	touch weight bearing
Tx	transplant
U&E	urea and electrolytes
UAO	upper airway obstruction
UAS	upper abdominal surgery
UL	upper limb/upper lobe
URTI	upper respiratory tract infection
USS	ultrasound scan
UTI	urinary tract infection
V	ventilation
V_A	alveolar ventilation/alveolar volume
VAD	ventricular assist device
VAS	visual analogue scale
VATS	video-assisted thoracoscopy surgery
VBG	venous blood gas
VC	vital capacity/volume control
V_E	minute ventilation
VE	ventricular ectopics
VEGF	vascular endothelial growth factor
VER	visual evoked response
VF	ventricular fibrillation/vocal fremitus
V/P shunt	ventricular peritoneal shunt
V/Q	ventilation/perfusion ratio
VR	vocal resonance
VRE	vancomycin-resistant enterococcus
VSD	ventricular septal defect
V_T	tidal volume
VT	ventricular tachycardia
WBC	white blood count
WCC	white cell count
WOB	work of breathing
W/R	ward round

Prefixes and suffixes

Prefix/suffix	Definition	Example
adeno-	gland	adenoma
-aemia	blood	hyperglycaemia
-algia	pain	neuralgia
angio-	vessel	angiogram
ante-	before	antenatal
arteri-	artery	arteriosclerosis
arthro-	joint	arthroscopy
-asis	condition	homeostasis
atel-	imperfect	atelectasis
auto-	self	autoimmunity
baro-	pressure	barotrauma
brachi-	arm	brachial artery
brady-	slow	bradycardia
carcin-	cancer	carcinogen
carpo-	wrist	carpal tunnel
cephal-	head	cephalad
chondro-	cartilage	chondromalacia
contra-	against	contraindicated
costo-	rib	costochondral junction
cranio-	skull	craniotomy
cut-	skin	cutaneous
cryo-	cold	cryotherapy
derm-	skin	dermatome
dys-	difficult	dyspnoea
-ectasis	dilatation	bronchiectasis
ecto-	outside	ectoplasm
-ectomy	excision	appendectomy
encephalo-	brain	encephalitis
endo-	within	endochondral
erythro-	red	erythrocyte
gastro-	stomach	gastroenteritis
haem-	blood	haematoma

Prefix/suffix	Definition	Example
hepato-	liver	hepatectomy
hyper-	excessive	hyperactive
hypo-	deficiency	hypoxaemia
idio-	one's own	idiopathic
iso-	equal	isotonic
-itis	inflammation	tendinitis
-lysis	breakdown	autolysis
-malacia	softening	osteomalacia
-megalo	enlarged	cardiomegaly
myo-	muscle	myotonic
nephro-	kidney	nephritis
oculo-	eyes	monocular
oligo-	deficiency	oliguria
-oma	tumour	lymphoma
-osis	state, condition	nephrosis
osteo-	bone	osteolysis
-penia	deficiency	thrombocytopenia
-plasia	formation	hyperplasia
-plasty	moulding	rhinoplasty
-plegia	paralysis	hemiplegia
poly-	many	polymyositis
pseud-	false	pseudoplegia
rhino-	nose	rhinitis
-rrhagia	abnormal flow	haemorrhage
sarco-	flesh	sarcoma
sclero-	hardening	scleroderma
somat-	body	somatic
spondyl-	vertebrae	spondylosis
-stasis	stagnation	haemostasis
steno-	narrow	stenosis
-stomy	surgical opening	colostomy
supra-	above	suprapubic
tachy-	swift	tachycardia
thrombo-	clot	thrombolytic
-tomy	incision	gastrostomy

Conversions and units

Lb/kg

lb	kg
1	0.45
2	0.91
3	1.36
4	1.81
5	2.27
6	2.72
7	3.18
8	3.63
9	4.08
10	4.54
11	4.99
12	5.44
13	5.90
14	6.35

Stones/kg

stones	kg
1	6.35
2	12.70
3	19.05
4	25.40
5	31.75
6	38.10
7	44.45
8	50.80
9	57.15
10	63.50
11	69.85
12	76.20
13	82.55

stones	kg
14	88.90
15	95.25
16	101.60
17	107.95
18	114.30

Mass

1 kilogramme (kg) = 2.205 pounds (lb)
1 pound (lb) = 454 milligrams (mg)
= 16 ounces (oz)
1 oz = 28.35 grams (g)

Length

1 inch (in) = 2.54 centimetres (cm)
1 metre (m) = 3.281 feet (ft)
= 39.37 in
1 foot (ft) = 30.48 cm
= 12 in

Volume

1 litre (L) = 1000 millilitres (ml)
1 pint ≈ 568 ml

Pressure

1 millimetre of mercury (mmHg) = 0.133 kilopascal (kPa)
1 kilopascal (kPa) = 7.5 mmHg

Physiotherapy management of the spontaneously breathing, acutely breathless patient

THE BREATHLESS PATIENT

↓

Assessment to identify cause: ←

→ **Respiratory** – amenable to physiotherapy

or

→ **Other** – Cardiac → **Liaise with medical staff**
- Renal
- Metabolic
- Neurological

Atelectasis	Bronchospasm	Sputum retention	Consolidation	Hypoxaemia	Pain	↑ Work of breathing	↓ Exercise tolerance
↓ SaO_2 Auscultation Percussion note CXR ABGs Thoracic expansion	↓ SaO_2 Auscultation ↓ PEFR CXR ABGs Breathing pattern	↓ SaO_2 Auscultation ↓ Sputum production Cough ABGs CXR Colour	↓ SaO_2 Percussion note Auscultation CXR ABGs	NB consider $PaCO_2$ ↓ SaO_2 ABGs Colour CXR Level of consciousness	↓ SaO_2 ABGs Cough Pain score	↓ SaO_2 Breathing pattern ABGs Cough	↓ SaO_2 ↓ Shuttle walk ↓ Borg Scale ABGs ↓ VAS

↓

Consider appropriate treatment *NB Patients may have a combination of the above problems*

Atelectasis	Bronchospasm	Sputum retention	Consolidation	Hypoxaemia	Pain	↑ Work of breathing	↓ Exercise tolerance
Mobilization Positioning to maximize – FRC – V/Q ACBT with inspiratory holds and sniffs Assisted ventilation – IPPB – CPAP – NIPPV	Positioning Breathing control Bronchodilator Therapy PEFR Neurophysiological facilitation techniques	Humidification NaCl nebulizers ↑ Hydration ACBT in appropriate positions Manual techniques Assisted cough IPPB Suction Mobilization	Positioning to maximize V/Q Humidification ↑ Hydration Observe	Oxygen therapy Positioning to maximize V/Q Assisted ventilation – IPPB – CPAP – NIPPV	Liaise with medical staff re: Pain control Positioning Wound support TENS Entonox	Positioning Breathing control Assisted ventilation – IPPB – CPAP – NIPPV Neurophysiological facilitation techniques	Breathing control Mobilization with O_2 Individualized exercise programme

↓

Select and apply treatment

↓

Evaluate outcome of treatment

↓

Improvement in subjective and objective markers → **Effective treatment** → **Continue with treatment plan**

No improvement or deterioration in subjective and objective markers → **Ineffective treatment** → **Reassess**

Figure A.1 Physiotherapy management of the spontaneously breathing, acutely breathless patient. With permission of the Association of Chartered Physiotherapists in Respiratory Care.

Adult basic life support (Resuscitation Council (UK) 2000, with permission)

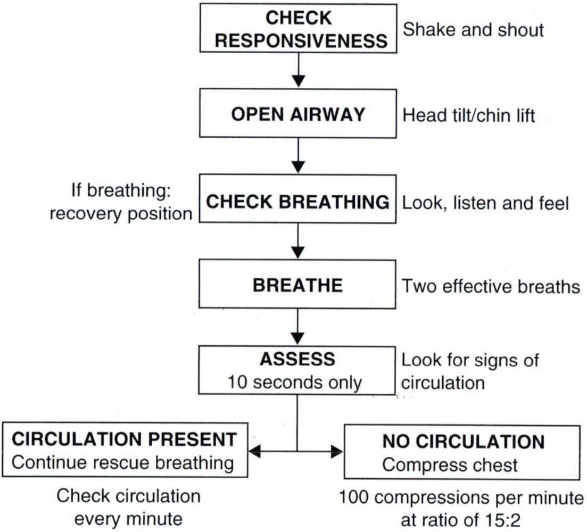

Send or go for help as soon as possible according to the guidelines

Resuscitation Guidelines 2000
Resuscitation Council (UK) www.resus.org.uk

Figure A.2 Adult basic life support.

Paediatric basic life support (Resuscitation Council (UK) 2000, with permission)

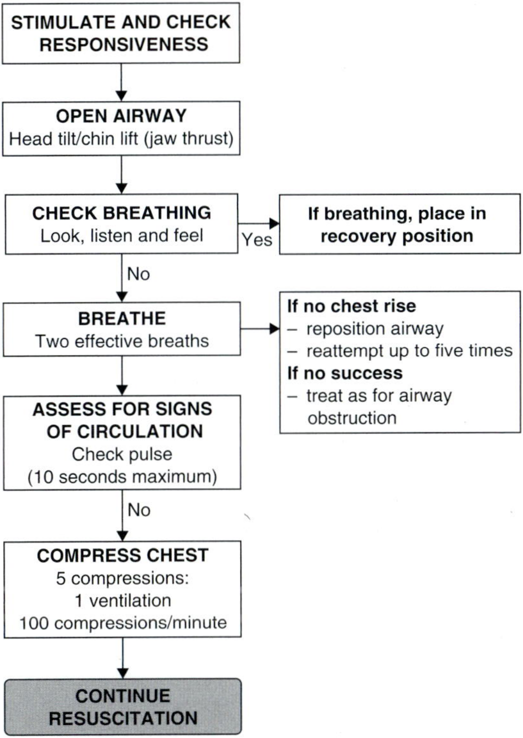

Resuscitation Guidelines 2000
Resuscitation Council (UK) www.resus.org.uk

Figure A.3 Paediatric basic life support.

Laboratory values (Brooker 2002)

Biochemistry

Alanine aminotransferase (ALT)	10–40 U/L
Albumin	36–47 g/L
Alkaline phosphatase	40–125 U/L
Amylase	90–300 U/L
Aspartate aminotransferase (AST)	10–35 U/L
Bicarbonate (arterial)	22–28 mmol/L
Bilirubin (total)	2–17 μmol/L
Caeruloplasmin	150–600 mg/L
Calcium	2.1–2.6 mmol/L
Chloride	95–105 mmol/L
Cholesterol (total)	Desirable level <5.2 mmol/L
Cholesterol (HDL)	
Men	0.5–1.6 mmol/L
Women	0.6–1.9 mmol/L
Copper	13–24 μmol/L
Creatine kinase (total)	
Men	30–200 U/L
Women	30–150 U/L
Creatinine	55–150 μmol/L
Globulins	24–37 g/L
Glucose	3.6–5.8 mmol/L
Iron	
Men	14–32 μmol/L
Women	10–28 μmol/L
Lactate (arterial)	0.3–1.4 mmol/L
Lactate dehydrogenase (total)	230–460 U/L
Magnesium	0.7–1.0 mmol/L
Osmolality	275–290 mmol/kg
Phosphate (fasting)	0.8–1.4 mmol/L
Potassium (serum)	3.6–5.0 mmol/L
Protein (total)	60–80 g/L

Sodium	136–145 mmol/L
Transferrin	2–4 g/L
Urea	2.5–6.5 mmol/L
Vitamin A	0.7–3.5 μmol/L
Vitamin C	23–57 μmol/L
Zinc	11–22 μmol/L

Haematology

Activated partial thromboplastin time (APTT)	30–40 sec
Bleeding time (Ivy)	2–8 min
Erythrocyte sedimentation rate (ESR)	
Adult men	1–10 mm/h
Adult women	3–15 mm/h
Fibrinogen	1.5–4.0 g/L
Folate (serum)	4–18 μg/L
Haemoglobin	
Men	130–180 g/L (13–18 g/dl)
Women	115–165 g/L (11.5–16.5 g/dl)
International normalized ratio (INR)	0.89–1.10
Mean cell haemoglobin (MCH)	27–32 pg
Mean cell haemoglobin concentration (MCHC)	30–35 g/dl
Mean cell volume (MCV)	78–95 fl
Packed cell volume (PCV or haematocrit)	
Men	0.40–0.54 (40–54%)
Women	0.35–0.47 (35–47%)
Platelets (thrombocytes)	$150–400 \times 10^9$/L
Prothrombin time (PT)	12–16 sec

Red cells	
Men	$4.5–6.5 \times 10^{12}$/L
Women	$3.85–5.30 \times 10^{12}$/L
White cell count (leucocytes)	$4.0–11.0 \times 10^{9}$/L

Values vary from laboratory to laboratory, depending on testing methods used. These reference ranges should be used as a guide only. All reference ranges apply to adults only; they may differ in children.

Reference

Brooker C 2002 Dictionary of nursing, 18th edn. Churchill Livingstone, Edinburgh

Index

B

C

D

E

F

G

H

I

J

K

L

N

O

P

Q

R

S

T

U

V

W

X

Z